The Socioeconomics of Health Care and the Practice of Urology

Guest Editor

KEVIN R. LOUGHLIN, MD, MBA

UROLOGIC CLINICS
OF NORTH AMERICA

www.urologic.theclinics.com

February 2009 • Volume 36 • Number 1

SAUNDERS an imprint of ELSEVIER, Inc.

W.B. SAUNDERS COMPANY
A Division of Elsevier Inc.

1600 John F. Kennedy Blvd. • Suite 1800 • Philadelphia, PA 19103-2899

http://www.theclinics.com

UROLOGIC CLINICS OF NORTH AMERICA Volume 36, Number 1
February 2009 ISSN 0094-0143, ISBN-13: 978-1-4377-0554-6, ISBN-10: 1-4377-0554-5

Editor: Kerry Holland
Developmental Editor: Donald Mumford

Urologic Clinics of North America (ISSN 0094-0143) is published quarterly by Elsevier Inc., 360 Park Avenue South, New York, NY 10010-1710. Months of issue are February, May, August, and November. Business and Editorial Offices: 1600 John F. Kennedy Blvd., Suite 1800, Philadelphia, PA 19103-2899. Periodicals postage paid at New York, NY and additional mailing offices. Subscription prices are $269.00 per year (US individuals), $429.00 per year (US institutions), $308.00 per year (Canadian individuals), $526.00 per year (Canadian institutions), $383.00 per year (foreign individuals), and $526.00 per year (foreign institutions). Foreign air speed delivery is included in all *Clinics* subscription prices. All prices are subject to change without notice. **POSTMASTER:** Send address changes to *Urologic Clinics of North America*, Elsevier Periodicals Customer Service, 11830 Westline Industrial Drive, St. Louis, MO 63146. Customer Service: 1-800-654-2452 (US). From outside the United States, call 1-314-453-7041. Fax: 1-314-453-5170. E-mail: JournalsCustomerServiceusa@elsevier.com (for print support) and JournalsOnlineSupport-usa@elsevier.com (for online support).

Reprints. For copies of 100 or more, of articles in this publication, please contact the Commercial Reprints Department, Elsevier Inc., 360 Park Avenue South, New York, New York 10010-1710. Tel.: 212-633-3813; Fax: 212-462-1935; E-mail: reprints@elsevier.com.

Urologic Clinics of North America is covered in MEDLINE/PubMed (*Index Medicus*), *Excerpta Medica, Current Contents/Clinical Medicine, Science Citation Index,* and *ISI/BIOMED*.

Printed and bound by CPI Group (UK) Ltd, Croydon, CR0 4YY
Transferred to Digital Print 2011

Contributors

GUEST EDITOR

KEVIN R. LOUGHLIN, MD, MBA
Senior Surgeon, Department of Urology,
Brigham and Women's Hospital; and Professor
of Surgery, Harvard Medical School, Boston,
Massachusetts

AUTHORS

ROBERT R. BAHNSON, MD, FACS
Dave Longaberger Chair in Urology, Professor
and Chairman, Department of Urology, Ohio
State University, Columbus, Ohio

R. ADAMS DUDLEY, MD, MBA
Associate Director for Research, Institute for
Health Policy Studies; and Associate Professor
of Medicine, Division of Pulmonary and Critical
Care Medicine, University of California,
San Francisco, California

LARS M. ELLISON, MD
Department of Urology, PenBay Medical
Center, Rockport, Maine

NEWT GINGRICH
Center for Health Transformation, The Gingrich
Group, Washington, District of Columbia

DAVID U. HIMMELSTEIN, MD
Associate Professor of Medicine, Harvard
Medical School, Department of Medicine,
Cambridge Hospital, Cambridge,
Massachusetts

BADRINATH M. KONETY, MD, MBA
Associate Professor and Vice Chairman,
Department of Urology; and Associate
Professor of Epidemiology and Biostatistics,
Department of Epidemiology and Biostatistics,
University of California, San Francisco,
California

LAURENCE J. KOTLIKOFF, PhD
Professor of Economics, Department of
Economics, Boston University, Boston,
Massachusetts

MARK S. LITWIN, MD, MPH
Professor of Urology and Health Services,
David Geffen School of Medicine and School of
Public Health, University of California; and
Jonsson Comprehensive Cancer Center,
University of California, Los Angeles, California

KEVIN R. LOUGHLIN, MD, MBA
Senior Surgeon, Department of Urology,
Brigham and Women's Hospital; and Professor
of Surgery, Harvard Medical School, Boston,
Massachusetts

DAVID MERRITT
Center for Health Transformation, The Gingrich
Group, Washington, District of Columbia

DAVID C. MILLER, MD, MPH
Assistant Professor of Urology and
Epidemiology, University of Michigan, Ann
Arbor, Michigan

CARL A. OLSSON, MD
Department of Urology, Columbia-
Presbyterian Hospital, College of Physicians
and Surgeons, Columbia University, New York,
New York

WILLIAM G. PLESTED III, MD
Immediate Past President, American Medical
Association, Chicago, Illinois

KIM F. RHOADS, MD, MPH
Assistant Professor of Surgery, Department of Surgery, Stanford University, Stanford; and Philip R. Lee Fellow in Health Policy, Institute for Health Policy Studies, University of California, San Francisco, California.

CHRISTOPHER S. SAIGAL, MD, MPH
Associate Professor of Urology, UCLA Department of Urology, David Geffen School of Medicine, University of California; and Jonsson Comprehensive Cancer Center, University of California, Los Angeles, California

STEVEN SCHLOSSBERG, MD, MBA
Professor of Urology, Eastern Virginia Medical School; Vice President, Medical Informatics, Sentara Healthcare, Norfolk, Virginia; and Vice Chairman, Health Policy, American Urologic Association, Linthicum, Maryland

LINDA M. DAIRIKI SHORTLIFFE, MD
Stanley McCormick Memorial Professor, Chair of the Department of Urology, Stanford University School of Medicine; Chief of Urology, Stanford University Medical Center; and Lucile Salter Packard Children's Hospital, Stanford, California

STEFFIE WOOLHANDLER, MD, MPH
Associate Professor of Medicine, Harvard Medical School, Department of Medicine, Cambridge Hospital, Cambridge, Massachusetts

MICHAEL J. ZINNER, MD
Surgeon-In-Chief, Brigham and Women's Hospital; and Mosely Professor of Surgery, Harvard Medical School, Boston, Massachusetts

Contents

THE HEALTHCARE LANDSCAPE: THE BIG PICTURE

The evolution of health care in America had its beginnings even before the founding of the nation. This article divides the evolution of American health care into six historical periods: (1) the charitable era, (2) the origins of medical education era, (3) the insurance era, (4) the government era, (5) the managed care era, and (6) the consumerism era.

The National Institute of Diabetes and Digestive and Kidney Diseases initiated the Urologic Diseases in America project in 2001 with the goal of quantifying the immense demographic burden of urologic diseases on the American public, in both human and financial terms. This effort was renewed in 2007 with the aim of expanding and deepening analyses of the epidemiology, costs, and quality of medical care in urology. This ongoing commitment recognizes the major public health impact of urologic conditions in the United States. A thoughtful policy response to these changes requires a thorough understanding of the health care resource use and clinical epidemiology relevant to urologic diseases in America. This article details major initial findings from the Urologic Diseases in America project with respect to the demographic impact of the most common benign, malignant, and pediatric urologic conditions.

The current American health care system is beyond repair. The problems of the health care system are delineated in this discussion. The current health care system needs to be replaced in its entirety with a new system that provides every American with first-rate, first-tier medicine and that doesn't drive our nation broke. The author describes a 10-point Medical Security System, which he proposes will address the problems of the current health care system.

The use of incentives to improve quality of care is spreading rapidly across the health care system. Public reporting (PR) and pay-for-performance (PFP) are two examples of incentive-based programs. Although conclusive level I evidence for the positive impacts of these PR and PFP is limited, individual states and the federal government have begun to adopt and pilot these programs for a variety of specific clinical conditions. This article reviews the principles of health care quality performance measurement; current reporting and pay-for-performance programs; and the most recent literature documenting positive, negative and future impacts of these types of programs on urologic practice.

The United States is in desperate need of health care reform. What has been brought to the table so far, however, has been insufficient. This article outlines a comprehensive change to health care delivery in the United States. If implemented, the author proposes that Americans will be healthier; more Americans will have health care; and costs can be greatly reduced.

The authors advocate a fundamental change in health care financing—national health insurance (NHI). NHI would reorient the way we pay for care, bringing the hundreds of billions now squandered on malignant bureaucracy back to the bedside. NHI could restore the physician-patient relationship, offer patients a free choice of physicians and hospitals, and free physicians from the hassles of insurance paperwork.

This article discusses the need for health care reform. The American Medical Association has devised a plan that would allow all Americans to obtain health care coverage. This article discusses that plan and advocates for physicians and patients to demand meaningful health care reform from lawmakers.

UROLOGIC PRACTICE: CURRENT ISSUES AND FUTURE PROSPECTS

Residency training in urologic surgery should change to an educational experience driven by outcomes instead of process. The needs analysis for curriculum modification has been completed and defines the competencies (enduring skills) of the complete physician. The challenge now rests with organizational leaders of urology to design programs that ensure the acquisition of these characteristics and conserve time and economic resources.

The process of certification, recertification, and maintenance of certification is mandated by the American Board of Urology as a member Board of the American Board of Medical Specialties. The history of maintenance of certification parallels that of private regulation of medical schools and postgraduate medical education (residency) and other nonmedical areas in which public trust is involved. Current trends in information technology that allow data gathering that measure medical practice and recognition of failure mandate that urologists practice with current knowledge. This will be documented in the maintenance of certification process.

The bulk of federal funding for medical research is delivered through the National Institutes of Health (NIH). Because federal funding is coordinated through the annual discretionary budget review process, the budget for NIH varies from year to year. Small changes in the rate of funding growth lead to significant problems for individual researchers and their supporting institutions. There is no single metric that serves as a surrogate to predict the appropriations process. This article begins with a history and physical examination of NIH. Next, the authors review the internal NIH priorities that continue to drive the funding process. Finally, the authors give a brief review of the impact congressionally mandated medical research programs have had on disease-specific funding.

With the changing environment for medical practice, physician practice models will continue to evolve. These "supergoups" create economies of scale, but their advantage is not only in the traditional economic sense. Practices with enough size are able to better meet the challenges of medical practice with increasing regulatory demands, explosion of clinical knowledge, quality and information technology initiatives, and an increasingly tight labor market. Smaller practices can adapt some of these strategies selectively. Depending on the topic, smaller practices should think differently about how to approach the challenges of practice.

The underpinning of medical practice has always been patient care and patient safety. The past several decades, however, have seen an erosion of the patient-doctor relationship. A number of factors have contributed to the ongoing medical malpractice crisis that continues in the United States. There are three social goals of malpractice litigation: to deter unsafe practices, to compensate persons injured through negligence, and to exact corrective justice. This article examines how well the current system achieves these goals.

GOAL STATEMENT

The goal of *Urologic Clinics of North America* is to keep practicing urologists and urology residents up to date with current clinical practice in urology by providing timely articles reviewing the state of the art in patient care.

ACCREDITATION

The *Urology Clinics of North America* is planned and implemented in accordance with the Essential Areas and Policies of the Accreditation Council for Continuing Medical Education (ACCME) through the joint sponsorship of the University of Virginia School of Medicine and Elsevier. The University of Virginia School of Medicine is accredited by the ACCME to provide continuing medical education for physicians.

The University of Virginia School of Medicine designates this educational activity for a maximum of *15 AMA PRA Category 1 Credits™*. Physicians should only claim credit commensurate with the extent of their participation in the activity.

The American Medical Association has determined that physicians not licensed in the US who participate in this CME activity are eligible for *15 AMA PRA Category 1 Credits™*.

Credit can be earned by reading the text material, taking the CME examination online at: http://www.theclinics.com/home/cme, and completing the evaluation. After taking the test, you will be required to review any and all incorrect answers. Following completion of the test and evaluation, your credit will be awarded and you may print your certificate.

FACULTY DISCLOSURE/CONFLICT OF INTEREST

The University of Virginia School of Medicine, as an ACCME accredited provider, endorses and strives to comply with the Accreditation Council for Continuing Medical Education (ACCME) Standards of Commercial Support, Commonwealth of Virginia statutes, University of Virginia policies and procedures, and associated federal and private regulations and guidelines on the need for disclosure and monitoring of proprietary and financial interests that may affect the scientific integrity and balance of content delivered in continuing medical education activities under our auspices.

The University of Virginia School of Medicine requires that all CME activities accredited through this institution be developed independently and be scientifically rigorous, balanced and objective in the presentation/discussion of its content, theories and practices.

All authors/editors participating in an accredited CME activity are expected to disclose to the readers relevant financial relationships with commercial entities occurring within the past 12 months (such as grants or research support, employee, consultant, stock holder, member of speakers bureau, etc.). The University of Virginia School of Medicine will employ appropriate mechanisms to resolve potential conflicts of interest to maintain the standards of fair and balanced education to the reader. Questions about specific strategies can be directed to the Office of Continuing Medical Education, University of Virginia School of Medicine, Charlottesville, Virginia.

The faculty and staff of the University of Virginia Office of Continuing Medical Education have no financial affiliations to disclose.

The authors/editors listed below have identified no professional or financial affiliations for themselves or their spouse/partner:

Robert R. Bahnson, MD, FACS; R. Adams Dudley, MD, MBA; Lars M. Ellison, MD; David U. Himmelstein, MD; Kerry K. Holland (Acquisitions Editor); Badrinath M. Konety, MD, MBA; Laurence J. Kotlikoff, PhD; Mark S. Litwin, MD, MPH; David C. Miller, MD, MPH; Carl A. Olsson, MD; William G. Plested III, MD; Kim F. Rhoads, MD, MPH; Christopher S. Saigal, MD, MPH; Steven M. Schlossberg, MD, MBA; William Steers, MD (Test Author); Steffie Woolhandler, MD, MPH; and, Michael J. Zinner, MD.

The authors/editors listed below have identified the following professional or financial affiliations for themselves or their spouse/partner:

Newt Gingrich is the founder of the Center for Health Transformation.
Kevin R. Loughlin, MD, MBA (Guest Editor) serves on the Advisory Board for Predictive Biosciences.
David Merritt is the project director of the Center for Health Transformation.
Linda M. Dairiki Shortliffe, MD is an independent director for Vivus.

Disclosure of Discussion of Non-FDA Approved Uses for Pharmaceutical Products and/or Medical Devices:
The University of Virginia School of Medicine, as an ACCME provider, requires that all faculty presenters identify and disclose any off label uses for pharmaceutical and medical device products. The University of Virginia School of Medicine recommends that each physician fully review all the available data on new products or procedures prior to clinical use.

TO ENROLL

To enroll in the *Urologic Clinics of North America* Continuing Medical Education program, call customer service at 1-800-654-2452 or visit us online at: http://www.theclinics.com/home/cme. The CME program is available to subscribers for an additional fee of $195.00.

Urologic Clinics of North America

THE CLINICS ARE NOW AVAILABLE ONLINE!

Access your subscription at:
www.theclinics.com

Preface

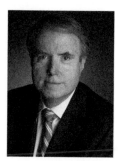

Kevin R. Loughlin, MD, MBA
Guest Editor

This is a unique issue for the *Urologic Clinics of North America*. For the first time, the *Clinics* have devoted an issue not to a clinical topic, but to the socioeconomics of health care. It is apparent that health care economics provide the underpinning of urologic practice for today and tomorrow. All of our clinical endeavors are dependent on the economic realties of the twenty-first century. We hope that this issue will elucidate some of the challenges that are facing patients, physicians, and society.

For the first time, we have authors who are physicians, but from several specialties other than urology. In addition, several of the authors are not physicians at all. These nonphysicians include an economist and the former speaker of the house of representatives.

Finally, the *Clinics* have only infrequently had issue dedications. However, it is indeed appropriate that this issue is dedicated to H. Logan Holtgrewe, who has contributed so much to clinical urology.

I have divided this issue into two major sections, "The Health Care Landscape: The Big Picture" and "Urologic Practice: Current Issues and Future Prospects." In the first section, the history and demographics of health care are reviewed, and following this, we have invited several authors to provide different proposals for health care reform. These proposals are followed by more parochial urologic issues that include residency training, certification and recertification, urologic research, practice management, and the impact of medical malpractice.

Kevin R. Loughlin, MD, MBA
Department of Urology
Brigham and Women's Hospital
45 Francis Street, ASB 11-3
Boston, MA 02115

E-mail address:
kloughlin@partners.org (K.R. Loughlin)

Urol Clin N Am 36 (2009) xi
doi:10.1016/j.ucl.2008.09.001
0094-0143/08/$ – see front matter © 2008 Elsevier Inc. All rights reserved.

urologic.theclinics.com

Dedication

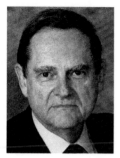

H. Logan Holtgrewe

Frannie Moore once said of Hartwell Harrison, "Hartwell Harrison is to urology as John Milton is to the English language. He didn't invent it, he merely refined and perfected it." The same can be said of H. Logan Holtgrewe regarding the practice of urology. Long before most Americans realized the impending health care crisis, Logan was on the front lines trying to achieve a system in which patient care was paramount and quality and efficiency were enhanced to create greater value.

One of the true characteristics of genius is vision; above all else, Logan was a visionary.

He initiated the Health Policy Council of the AUA and served as President of the AUA and the Board of Urology. He was also the recipient of the AUA's highest honor, the Ramon Guiteras Award.

It gives me great personal pleasure to dedicate this issue of the *Urologic Clinics of North America*, which is devoted to the socioeconomics of health care, to H. Logan Holtgrewe. Let this serve as recognition of the debt that we all owe to him and the great esteem in which he is held.

Kevin R. Loughlin, MD, MBA

Urol Clin N Am 36 (2009) xiii
doi:10.1016/j.ucl.2008.09.002

urologic.theclinics.com

The Evolution of Health Care in America

Michael J. Zinner, MD, Kevin R. Loughlin, MD, MBA*

KEYWORDS

• Evolution • Health care • America

The evolution of health care in America had its beginnings even before the founding of the nation. For the purposes of this article, the evolution of American health care is divided into six historical periods: (1) the charitable era, (2) the origins of medical education era, (3) the insurance era, (4) the government era, (5) the managed care era, and (6) the consumerism era. A summary of the timeframes of these eras appears in **Fig. 1**.

THE CHARITABLE ERA

In the precolonial and colonial era there was no organized health care in North America. Hospitals were formed out of public alms houses and care was delivered as a charitable endeavor. After public facilities were begun, religious orders formed hospitals for indigent care. The wealthy could afford to be seen at home. The first hospital founded in this era was the Pennsylvania Hospital, in Philadelphia, in 1752 (**Fig. 2**). This was followed by New York Hospital in 1791, the Boston Dispensary in 1796, and the Massachusetts General Hospital in 1811. During this period, medical schools began by associating with existing hospitals. Most of the schools were proprietary and to a large extent diploma mills.

THE EDUCATIONAL ERA: THE ORIGINS OF AMERICAN MEDICAL EDUCATION

Medical school education as it is known today was slow to evolve. The medical school of the University of Pennsylvania was founded in 1765, soon followed by King's College, later to become the College of Physicians and Surgeons, in 1768. Harvard Medical School was started in 1782. For much of the nineteenth century medical school education was poorly regulated and there was no standardized, agreed on curriculum for either undergraduate or postgraduate medical education.

In 1889, the Johns Hopkins Hospital was founded and the influence of Halsted, Osler, and the other Hopkins faculty provided the underpinnings for the modern residency training model. Residency education was based on a full-time faculty staff model with increasing responsibility throughout training and a final year of independence.

As great an influence as Hopkins was on the evolution of postgraduate medical education, the Flexner report of 1910 initiated an even greater change on undergraduate medical school education.[1] In 1904, the American Medical Association created the Council on Medical Education, whose objective was to restructure American medical education. At this time, there was no universal agreement on the requirements for entrance into medical school, nor was there a standardized medical school curriculum. Many medical schools were "proprietary," owned by one or more doctors, unaffiliated with a university, and run to make a profit.[1] The Council on Medical Education adopted two standards: minimal education requirements for medical school admission, and medical school education should be composed of 2 years of training in human anatomy and physiology followed by 2 years of clinical work in a teaching hospital.

In 1910, Abraham Flexner, a professional educator, was commissioned by the Carnegie Foundation to assess medical school education. Flexner visited all 155 schools in North America and found a wide divergence in their curricula and requirements for admission and graduation.

Department of Urology, Brigham and Women's Hospital, 45 Francis Street, ASB 11-3, Boston, MA 02115, USA
* Corresponding author.
E-mail address: kloughlin@partners.org (K.R. Loughlin).

Urol Clin N Am 36 (2009) 1–10
doi:10.1016/j.ucl.2008.08.005

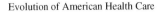

Evolution of American Health Care

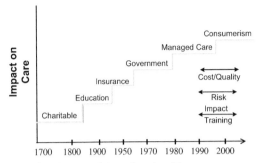

Fig. 1. The six eras of American health care.

After his extensive study, Flexner made the following recommendations in his report:

1. Medical school admission should require, at a minimum, a high school diploma and at least 2 years of college or university study. Before the Flexner Report, only 16 of the 155 medical schools in the United States and Canada required at least 2 years of university study for admission.
2. The length of medical school education should be 4 years and its content should follow the Council on Medical Education guidelines of 1905.
3. Proprietary medical schools should either close or be incorporated into existing universities.

The impact of the Flexner Report on medical school education and training cannot be overestimated. In 1904, there were 160 medical degree granting institutions with more than 28,0000 students in the United States and Canada. By 1920, there were only 85 institutions with only 13,800 students, and by 1935 there were only 66 medical schools in the United States.[1] Of these 66 surviving medical schools, 57 were part of a university.

It was this revolution in medical school and postgraduate medical education that occurred in the later nineteenth and early twentieth century that

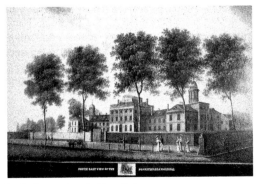

Fig. 2. Pennsylvania Hospital.

laid the foundation for the changes in health care organization and delivery that followed later in the twentieth century.

THE INSURANCE ERA

Although insurance has been around for centuries, it was not applied to medical care until the first half of the twentieth century. In 1929, a group of teachers in Dallas, Texas, contracted with Baylor Hospital for medical services in exchange for a monthly fee.

It was Sidney R. Garfield, however, a young surgeon, who really laid the foundation for prepaid health insurance in 1933. Garfield saw thousands of men involved in building the Los Angeles Aqueduct and saw an opportunity to provide health care to those workers. He borrowed money to build Contractors General Hospital near a small town called Desert Center in the middle of the Mohave Desert. Garfield had trouble getting insurance companies to pay the medical expenses of the workers, however, and soon both the hospital and Garfield were running into financial trouble. At that point, Harold Hatch, an insurance agent, approached Garfield with the idea that insurance companies pay a fixed amount per day, per covered worker, up front. For 5 cents per day, workers received this new form of health coverage.

In 1938, the industrialist Henry J. Kaiser and his son, Edgar, were building the Grand Coulee Dam in Washington state and the labor unions were dissatisfied with the fee-for-service care being provided to the 10,000 workers and their families because it was relatively expensive and beyond what many workers could afford. Edgar Kaiser invited Dr. Garfield to form a medical group to provide health care to the workers at a cost of 7 cents per day to be prepaid by the company. This coverage was soon expanded to include the workers' wives and children. Four years later, during World War II, Henry Kaiser expanded the Garfield model to his wartime shipyards and then to the Kaiser steel mills in Fontana, in Southern California. Kaiser then bought his own hospital in Oakland and the name Permanente was adopted, picked by Henry Kaiser's first wife, Bess, because of her love of the Permanente Creek that flows year round on the San Francisco peninsula.

Parallel to the genesis of the Kaiser-Permanente system was the development of the early Blue Cross insurance plans. In 1932, the American Hospital Association introduced the first Blue Cross plan that was a prepayment model to hospitals to provide care to enrolled patients. The early Blue Cross plans were nonprofits that received a tax break enabling them to keep premiums low. Blue Shield plans, which were contracted to cover physicians' services, soon followed.

During World War II, there were strict wage and price controls. Strong unions bargained for better benefit packages, including tax-free, employer-sponsored health insurance. Because employers could not, under law, increase wages, they attracted workers by providing better benefit packages, including health care. This laid the foundation for the rapid expansion of employer-subsidized health care in the post–World War II era.

THE GOVERNMENT ERA

The origins of the rationale for government involvement in health care delivery can be traced to the 1940s. In 1943, the Wagner-Murray-Dingell Bill was proposed, which provided for comprehensive health care delivery under the Social Security system; however, the legislation was never approved by Congress. On November 19, 1945, just 7 months after taking office, Truman gave a speech before Congress during which he called for the creation of a national health insurance fund to be administered by the federal government. The fund would be open to all Americans, but would remain optional and participants would pay monthly fees for enrolment.

In part because of Truman's endorsement of the role of the federal government in medical care, the Hill-Burton Act was passed in 1946. This bill was designed to provide federal grants to improve the infrastructure of the nation's hospital system. It provided for the construction and improvement of hospital facilities to achieve a goal of 4.5 beds per 1000 people.[1]

In 1960, Congress passed the Kerr-Mills Act or Medical Assistance for the Aged. This was a means-tested program that contributed federal funds to state-run medical assistance programs for the elderly who could not afford adequate medical care. One major flaw of the program was that five states received 90% of the funds.[2] The Kerr-Mills Act, however, provided the underpinning for the passage of the Medicare and Medicaid laws, which were passed in 1965. President Johnson signed the bill as part of his "Great Society" program and former president Truman was the first enrollee (**Fig. 3**). Since the inception of Medicare, the number of enrollees has increased from 19 million to 40 million and the expenditures for Medicare have increased faster than any other federal program.[3] It is estimated that by 2030 Medicare will serve 68 million people or one in five Americans and will account for 4.4% of the gross domestic product.[4]

In the 1980s Medicare changed from a cost-based system of payment to hospitals and physicians to a system where payments are predetermined with hospitals receiving a flat rate based on diagnosis.[3] Hospital payments were capitated using diagnostic-related group payments. Hsiao and coworkers[4] with the support of the Health Care Financing Administration introduced the resource-based relative value scale, which determined input by time spent, intensity of work, practice costs, and the costs for advanced training.[4]

Medicaid was also passed in 1965 under Title XIX of the Social Security Act and provided for federal financial assistance to states that operated approved medical assistance plans.[5] Medicaid is a state administered program and each state sets its own guidelines regarding eligibility and services. In 2005, there were 53 million people enrolled in Medicaid and the program cost over $300 billion in federal and state spending. Rosenbaum[6] identified the fundamental reason that Medicaid spending is difficult, if not impossible,

Evolution of Health Care
Government Era

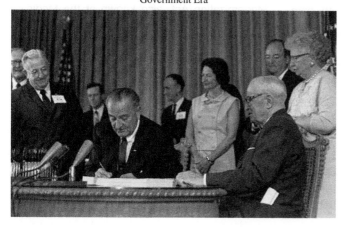

Fig. 3. President Johnson signing the Medicare legislation in 1965 as ex-president Truman looks on.

Table 1	
Federal initiatives in health care delivery	
1943	Wagner-Murray-Dingell bill
1945	President Truman endorses national health insurance
1946	Hill-Burton Act
1960	Kerr-Mills Act
1965	Medicare and Medicaid laws passed
1993	Clinton plan
1996	Kassebaum-Kennedy Act
2003	Medicare Modernization Act

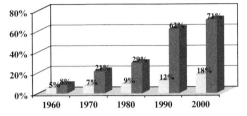

Health care costs as a percent of GNP

Health care costs as a percent of pretax corporate profits

Fig. 4. Commercial operations marketing forces. Impact of rising health care costs.

to harness when he stated "Federal financing of state Medicaid plans is open-ended. Each participating state is entitled to payments up to a federally approved percentage of state expenditures, and there is no limit on total payments to any state.....With federal contributions limited only by the size of state programs, Medicaid encourages its own growth and expansion."

In 1993, Clinton became president and a major component of his legislature agenda was the implementation of a national health care program. He appointed his wife, Hillary Rodman Clinton, as the major advocate of its presentation to Congress. It is noteworthy that there was little if any consultation with physicians as to the formulation and planning of what became known as the Clinton Plan.

Despite its introduction with a great deal of publicity, the Clinton Plan never achieved Congressional approval. This was caused by several factors. First, it was not managed well politically and it came to be viewed as a highly partisan rather than a bipartisan initiative. Second, the public appetite for an all-inclusive national health care program was lacking. Although the remainder of the 1990s would witness further modifications in the Medicare and Medicaid programs, there was no emergence of a federally based all inconclusive national health care system.[7] Notable, however, was the 1996 legislation sponsored by Senators Kassebaum and Kennedy, which included a provision for the creation of up to 665,000 medical savings accounts to be available to the self-employed and firms with less than 50 employees.

Concurrent with increased care delivery were the soaring costs of prescription drugs. In 1999, the cost of prescription drugs in the United Stats reached $100 billion, an increase of 16.9%.[8] Total national spending on prescription drugs doubled from 1995 to 2000 and tripled from 1990 to 2000.[9] Americans have demonstrated an increased reliance on drugs, caused in part by the aging of the population and new drug discovery.[10] The average number of retail prescriptions per American per year increased from 8.3 in 1995 to 10.5 in 2000.[10] The increase in the elderly was even more pronounced with the number of prescriptions increasing from 19.6 per individual per year in 1992, to 28.5 in 2000, to 34.4 in 2005, and projected to rise to 38.5 in 2010.[11]

As a political response to this specific component of rising health care costs, Congress passed the Medicare Prescription Drug, Improvement and Modernization Act, also known at the Medicare

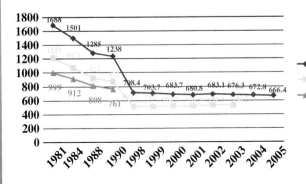

Fig. 5. Los Angeles use: hospital days. (*Data from* AHA Hospital Statistics, 2007 health forum.)

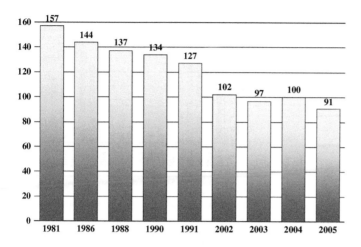

Fig. 6. Los Angeles use: number of hospitals. (*Data from* AHA Hospital Statistics, 2007; United States Statistical Abstract, 1991.)

Modernization Act or Medicare Part D, late in 2003. The passage of this bill was a major legislative initiative of President Bush and the original estimate of the cost was approximately $400 billion over 10 years. Within months of passage, however, the cost estimate was adjusted upward to $534 billion by Medicare chief McClellan.[12] Subsequent analyses have suggested that the true cost of this drug benefit may reach $1.2 trillion.[13]

The past six decades have witnessed legislation that has markedly increased federal participation and government control of health care delivery. The major legislation passed during this period is summarized in **Table 1**.

THE MANAGED CARE ERA

Parallel to this period of increased federal intrusion into health care was an inexorable rise in health care costs. **Fig. 4** summarizes the increasing health care costs as a percent of the Gross National Product and contrasts that with health care costs as a percent of pretax corporate profits. These economic forces provided the impetus for the managed care era. This so called "managed

care" era was really an attempt to mange costs. It was characterized by the conversion of not-for-profit health plans to investor owned-for-profit health plans. It was designed to remove the excesses from the health care system with capitation and commodity pricing to restrain costs.

The first pressure of the managed care era was to reduce the length of stay in hospitals. Los Angeles serves as a good example of this phenomenon. The dramatic decline of hospitals days per 1000 over the last two decades of the twentieth century in Los Angeles appears in **Fig. 5**. Similar trends were observed throughout the country.

The second pressure of the managed care era was to reduce the number of hospitals. This phenomenon also occurred and the significant decline in hospitals resulted in a dramatic decline in in-patient hospital beds. The trends in the number of hospitals in Los Angeles and Massachusetts appear in **Figs. 6** and **7**.

These constraints were a direct attempt to limit health care costs, and to a large extent they achieved that goal. **Fig. 8** displays the dramatic decrease in the annual growth rates for health insurance premiums between 1988 and 1996.

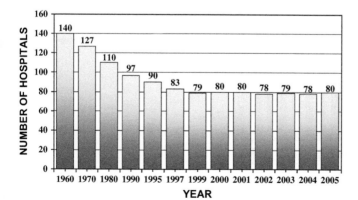

Fig. 7. Massachusetts acute care hospitals, 1960–2005. (*Data from* AHA Hospital Statistics, 2007.)

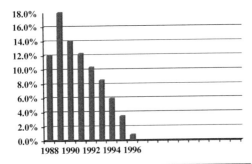

Fig. 8. Annual growth rates for health insurance premiums, 1988–1996. (*Data from* Kaiser Family Foundation/Health Research and Educational Trust.)

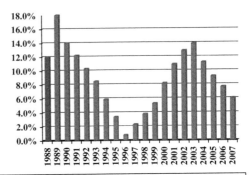

Fig. 9. Annual growth rates for health insurance premiums, 1998–2007. Data based on family of four. (*Data from* Kaiser Family Foundation/Health Research and Educational Trust.)

Managed care proved not to be the panacea for the health care crisis that some initially perceived it to be. Patient choice and access emerged as major issues. Throughout the era of managed care there was increasing disenchantment by both enrollees and providers. Enrollees were increasingly frustrated by gate keepers, use review, and restriction or lack of choice of physician. Physicians were unhappy because of what they perceived as increasing interference in the doctor-patient relationship. In addition, it was evident that capitation shifted the financial risk from the insurer to the provider.[14]

Robinson[15] provided a cogent analysis as to some of the reasons why managed care unraveled when he observed, "Controlling health care costs behind the scenes is difficult even in the most propitious circumstances; it became volatile in the context of reports of excessive profits, bureaucratic hassle and exorbitant executive earnings."

He further commented, "The fundamental flaw of managed care, in retrospect, was that it sought to navigate the tensions between limited resources and unlimited expectations without explaining exactly how it was so doing."[15] Iglehart[16] provided further analysis when he cautioned, "If physicians feel alienated from the system because they genuinely believe they are being dealt with unfairly, the damage to payers, patients and providers will be substantial, since no system can be stronger than the human interactions at its center."

THE CONSUMER ERA

As the disenchantment with managed care increased, patients became more concerned

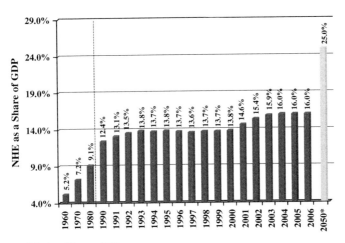

* Projected for year 2050

Fig. 10. National health expenditures as share of gross domestic product, 1960–2006. (*Data from* Kaiser Family Foundation: Health Care Marketplace Project 2007.)

The National Healthcare Expenditures (NHE) is projected to nearly double between 2006 and 2015, with healthcare expected to account for 20 percent of GDP by 2015.

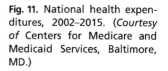

Fig. 11. National health expenditures, 2002–2015. (*Courtesy of* Centers for Medicare and Medicaid Services, Baltimore, MD.)

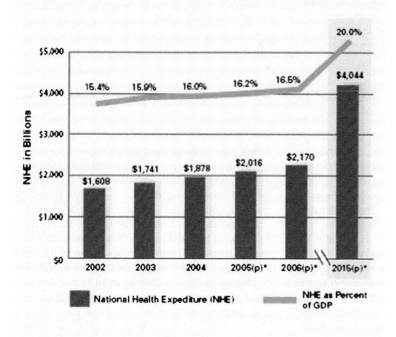

*Projected by Centers for Medicare and Medicaid Services.

with the quality and not just the cost of care. The concept of value emerged.

The first consequences of the failure of the managed care era were that premiums began to rise. As displayed in **Fig. 9**, starting in the late 1990s, the growth rates of insurance premiums increased fairly rapidly. The overall national expenditures as expressed as percentage of the gross domestic product also continued to increase (**Fig. 10**). This trend is projected to continue and the Centers for Medicare and Medical Services project that health care spending will reach 20% of the gross domestic product by 2015 (**Fig. 11**). Compounding this trend is the aging of the population. As displayed in **Fig. 12**, projections estimate that the over age 65 population will approximately double in the next 20 years.

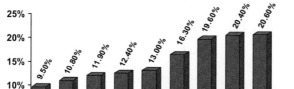

Fig. 12. Aging population. (*Data from* US census bureau.)

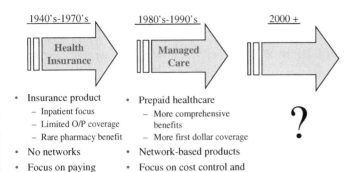

Fig. 13. Evolution of paying for care.

If one reflects on the economics of American health care in the past half century or so, one observes an evolution from private insurance to government programs and to managed care (**Figs. 13 and 14**). The question is, what does the future hold?

As health care costs continued to rise and the economy stalled, employers sought to unload more of the burden of health care expenses back to the employee.[17] The dilemma of rising health care costs went beyond the employer-employee relationship. The costs of health care were passed on to the consumer, as General Motors estimated that $1400 of the price of each vehicle was caused by employee medical costs.[18]

If one speculates on the future course of the consumerism era it seems that purchasers (companies and government) want to shift the risk to patients. Purchasers want transparency of costs and quality and safety. Patients, in effect, have become the "purchaser."

In 1999, the Institute of Medicine published its landmark report, *To Err is Human: Building a Safer Health System*. Many credit this publication as

giving rise to the patient safety movement. In the ensuring years there was more and more transparency as hospitals both voluntarily and by mandate began to publish safety data.[19] Safety alone does not equal quality, but it is an important element.

Strategies to enhance patient safety do not have to increase the cost of care. If done correctly they should decrease costs and add value to the consumer. Gawande[20] has advocated the application of checklists, which are common in aviation and other nonmedical industries, to improve outcomes and patient safety in an intensive care setting. Such checklists have potentially wide applications in many aspects of medical care, however, and have been applied to preoperative preparation immediately before commencing surgery in the operating room.[21]

Porter and Teisberg[22] have expanded on the concept of value in health care delivery. They remind the reader that increased costs per se do not impugn value and state "Success can only be measured by the value delivered per dollar spent. Spending more is not necessarily a problem, the question is whether Americans are getting

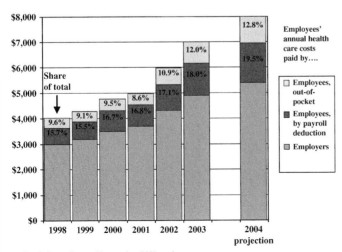

Fig. 14. Employee's annual health care costs. (*Adapted from* Freudenheim M. Workers feel pinch of rising health costs. New York Times, October 22, 2003.)

their money's worth. Americans collectively spend more on computers than they did ten years ago, for instance, because today's computers offer much greater value."

Porter and Teisberg[22] outline the principles of value-based competition, which is a positive-sum competition in which all system participants can benefit: when providers win by delivering superior care more efficiently, patients, employers, and insurers win. When health plans help patients and referring physicians make better choices and reward excellent care, providers benefit. They further state that when providers and health care plans and physicians compete to achieve the best medical outcomes for patients, they pursue the aims that attracted them to the profession in the first place.

Porter and Teisberg[22] outline eight principles that should be the guides for value-based competition in health care. These principles are summarized in **Box 1**. A detailed discussion of these principles is beyond the scope of this article, but is clear that the concept of "value" so prevalent in other industries is making its entrance into health care delivery.

PATIENT RESPONSIBILITY

As the era of consumerism progresses, it is important to acknowledge that the patient has an

> **Box 1**
> **Principles of value-based competition**
>
> 1. The focus should be on value for patients, not just lowering costs.
> 2. Competition must be based on results.
> 3. Competition should center on medical conditions over the full cycle of care.
> 4. High quality care should be less costly.
> 5. Value must be driven by provider experience, scale and learning at the medical condition.
> 6. Competition should be regional and national, not just local.
> 7. Results information to support value-based competition must be widely available.
> 8. Innovations that increase value must be strongly rewarded.
>
> *From* Porter ME, Teisberg EO. Redefining health care: creating value-based competition on results. Boston: Harvard Business School; 2006. p. 100; with permission.

important responsibility for his or her own health. Far too little emphasis has been placed by either federal or private sector payors on the responsibility of the patient to maintain good health habits.

Over a half century ago, Luther Terry, then the Surgeon-General of the United States, announced the link between tobacco smoking and lung

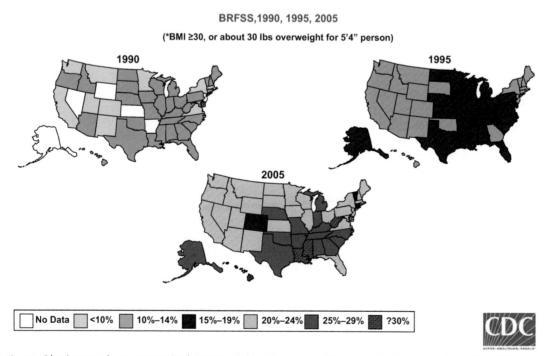

Fig. 15. Obesity trends among United States adults. (*Courtesy of* Behavioral Risk Factor Surveillance System, Centers for Disease Control and Prevention, Atlanta, GA.)

cancer. Since that time a preponderance of evidence has shown the harmful effects of tobacco on a myriad of disease processes. The President's Cancer Panel estimates that 14 million Americans have died prematurely because of smoking and that tobacco use accounts for 30% of all cancer deaths. Despite this persuasive evidence, 21% of Americans still smoke.

The obesity epidemic continues unabated in the United States, so much so that expensive bariatric surgery has emerged as a surgical subspecialty. If one defines obesity as a body mass index greater than 30 or about 30 lb overweight for a 5-ft 4-in person, one can review data from the Centers for Disease Control and Prevention that illustrate the inexorable obesity trend in the United States. According to the Centers for Disease Control and Prevention data, in 1990 no state had greater than 14% of their population defined as obese. By 1995, only 23 states still met this benchmark, with 27 states then having 20% or more of their population considered obese. In 2005, 45 states had greater than 20% of their population meet the obesity criteria. These data appear in **Fig. 15**.

If value is to be truly embraced as the sine qua non of this health care era, far greater personal responsibility needs to be placed on the patient. Bloche[23] recently observed, "If the United States is to come close to universal coverage, personal responsibility will need to play a larger role than it did in the mid-20th century welfare state... The new compact is likely to start with an enhanced sense of individual obligation-to eat sensibly, exercise regularly, avoid smoking and otherwise care for ourselves."

SUMMARY

A recent New York Times editorial communicated the urgency of the current health care crisis when it stated, "By now it should be clear that there is no silver bullet to restrain soaring health care costs. A wide range of contributing factors needs to be tackled simultaneously, with no guarantee they will have a substantial impact any time soon. In many cases, we do not have enough solid information to know how to cut costs without impairing quality."[11] What is clear is that it will require sacrifice and discipline from all involved in the health care industry to achieve the desired results: quality care of exceptional value for all Americans. What is even clearer is that the stakes are enormously high. If society fails to achieve these goals, the consequences are dire. If society succeeds, however, a health care system that is the paradigm for future generations will be achieved.

REFERENCES

1. Wikipedia. Available at: www.wikipedia.org. Accessed January 15, 2008.
2. Folland S, Goodman AC, Stano M. The economics of health and healthcare. 3rd edition. Upper Saddle River (NJ): Prentice Hall; 2001. p. 507.
3. Moon M. Medicare. N Engl J Med 2001;344(12): 928–31.
4. Hsiao WC, Dunn DL, Verrilli DK. Assessing the implementation of physician payment reform. N Engl J Med 1993;328(13):928–33.
5. Enthoven A, Kronick R. A consumer choice health plan for the 1990s: universal health insurance in a system designed to promote quality and economy. N Engl J Med 1989;320(2):94–101.
6. Rosenbaum S. Medicaid. N Engl J Med 2002;346(8): 635–40.
7. Loughlin KR. Urologists on a tightrope: do we have a net? J Urol 2003;170(6 Pt 1):2173–80.
8. Iglehart JK. Medicare and prescription drugs. N Engl J Med 2001;344(13):1010–5.
9. Pear R. Propelled by drug and hospital costs, health care spending surged in 2000. NY Times January 8, 2002. p. A14.
10. Levit K, Smith C, Cowan C, et al. Inflation spurs health spending in 2000. Health Aff 2002;21(1): 172–81.
11. Available at: familiesusa.org. Accessed January 15, 2008.
12. Boehlert E. Lies, bribes and hidden costs. Available at: Salon.com. Accessed April 5, 2004.
13. Connolly C, Allen M. Medicare drug benefit may cost $1.2 trillion. Washington Post February 9, 2005;A01.
14. Dudley RA, Luft HS. Managed care in transition. N Engl J Med 2001;344:1087.
15. Robinson JC. The end of managed care. JAMA 2001;285:2622.
16. Iglehart JK. The American healthcare system: introduction. N Engl J Med 1992;326:962.
17. Freudenheim M. Workers feel pinch of rising health costs. NY Times October 22, 2003.
18. Akst D. The hidden price tag for healthcare. NY Times December 12, 2004.
19. Kershaw S. In bid for transparency, New York City puts data on hospital errors online. NY Times September 7, 2007. p. A26.
20. Gawande A. The checklist, The New Yorker. December 10, 2007. p. 86–95.
21. Available at: indeltalearning.com. Accessed January 15, 2008.
22. Porter ME, Teisberg EO. Redefining health care: creating value-based competition on results. Boston: Harvard Business School Press; 2006. p. 100.
23. Bloche MG. Health care for all? N Engl J Med 2007; 357(12):1173.

The Demographic Burden of Urologic Diseases in America

David C. Miller, MD, MPH[a], Christopher S. Saigal, MD, MPH[b,c], Mark S. Litwin, MD, MPH[b,c,d],*

KEYWORDS

- Benign prostatic hyperplasia • Urinary incontinence
- Erectile dysfunction • Prostate cancer • Bladder cancer
- Hypospadias • Undescended testis
- Vesicoureteral reflux

The National Institute of Diabetes and Digestive and Kidney Diseases initiated the Urologic Diseases in America (UDA)[1] project in 2001 with the goal of quantifying the immense demographic burden of urologic diseases on the American public, in both human and financial terms (**Box 1**). This effort was renewed in 2007 with the aim of expanding and deepening analyses of the epidemiology, costs, and quality of medical care in urology. This ongoing commitment recognizes the major public health impact of urologic conditions in the United States. Urologic disorders occur from the earliest stages in development through the end of life. Many are chronic and affect individuals not by shortening survival, but by impairing quality of life. The economic impact of urologic diseases is often substantial for patients and families, employers, payers, and society at large (**Tables 1 and 2**). Moreover, physician practice and patient care-seeking behavior in urology have changed dramatically in response to a variety of financial and nonfinancial incentives in recent years. A thoughtful policy response to these changes requires a thorough understanding of the health care resource use and clinical epidemiology relevant to urologic diseases in America, particularly as society prepares for the large demographic shifts expected as the baby boom generation ages.

UDA analyses use multiple and diverse sources of epidemiologic and health services data to document one or more of the following trends for a broad spectrum of urologic disease: (1) demographic and secular trends in overall costs; (2) changes in physician practice patterns for diagnostic and therapeutic interventions; (3) changes in the specialty of treating physicians; (4) changes in the demographic characteristics of patients and treating physicians; and (5) demographic and secular trends in resource use, such as inpatient hospital resources, length of stay, outpatient physician and facility resources, use of pharmaceuticals and durable medical equipment, and availability and type of insurance coverage. Until the UDA project, no authoritative omnibus had compiled a comprehensive set of data analyses that synthesized information available from myriad national and regional sources across the public and private sectors in the United States. These sources, rich with epidemiologic and economic data on trends in the diagnosis and management of urologic diseases, were prodigiously tapped for a UDA compendium prepared by the University of California, Los Angeles, and RAND in 2007 (www.uda.niddk.nih.gov and www.udaonline.net). This article details major initial findings from the UDA project with respect to the demographic

This work was supported by award No. N01-DK-1-2460 from the National Institutes of Health.

[a] Departments of Urology and Epidemiology, University of Michigan, Ann Arbor, MI, USA
[b] Department of Urology, David Geffen School of Medicine, University of California, Los Angeles, CA, USA
[c] Department of Health Services, School of Public Health, University of California, Los Angeles, CA, USA
[d] Jonsson Comprehensive Cancer Center, University of California, Los Angeles, CA, USA
* Corresponding author.
E-mail address: mlitwin@mednet.ucla.edu (M.S. Litwin).

Prostate

Chronic and acute prostatitis

Benign prostatic hyperplasia

Prostate cancer

Bladder

Interstitial cystitis and painful bladder syndrome

Urinary incontinence in women

Urinary incontinence in men

Bladder cancer

Kidney

Urolithiasis

Ureteropelvic junction obstruction

Kidney cancer

Pediatrics

Vesicoureteral reflux

Undescended testis

Hypospadias

Ureterocele

Posterior urethral valves

Urinary tract infection in children

Urinary incontinence in children

Male Health

Infertility

Erectile dysfunction and Peyronie's disease

Urethral stricture

Testicular cancer

Infections

Urinary tract infection in women

Urinary tract infection in men

Sexually transmitted diseases

impact of the most common benign, malignant, and pediatric urologic conditions.

BENIGN UROLOGIC CONDITIONS
Benign Prostatic Hyperplasia

Benign prostatic hyperplasia (BPH), a chronic and often progressive condition, affects nearly three in four men by the seventh decade of life. Recognizing its clinical and public health significance, UDA investigators used a variety of data sources, including administrative data sets, large national health surveys, and community-based studies, to characterize the demographic burden of illness attributable to BPH and its associated medical care.

For an increasing number of men with BPH, the outpatient physician office represents the portal of entry into the health care system. Illustrating this trend with data from the National Ambulatory Medical Care Survey (NAMCS) and the National Hospital Ambulatory Medical Care Survey, an increase in the number of outpatient visits for BPH from 10,116 per 100,000 in 1994 to 14,473 per 100,000 in 2000 was observed (**Table 3**). During the same period, BPH-related emergency room visits decreased from 330 per 100,000 in 1994 to 218 per 100,000 in 2000.[2] Follow-up visits for imaging, prescriptions, and office-based surgical interventions are likely to be contributing factors to this trend.

Other UDA data sources allowed characterization of the clinical evaluations, medical therapies, and procedural interventions that accompany these outpatient visits. For instance, most urologists recommend medical therapy with α-blockers or 5-α-reductase inhibitors as first-line treatment for men with symptomatic BPH.[3] NAMCS data provide empiric support for this practice pattern.[2] Specifically, in 2000, 23% of prescriptions written at BPH-related outpatient visits were for the α-blockers, doxazosin and tamsulosin. That year, only 7.3% of BPH-related outpatient visits culminated in a prescription for the 5-α-reductase inhibitor, finasteride. The widespread use of these pharmacologic agents is supported by a broad clinical literature including the landmark National Institute of Diabetes and Digestive and Kidney Diseases–funded Medical Therapy of Prostatic Symptoms study, which demonstrated that combination therapy (α-blocker and 5-α-reductase inhibitor) was nearly twice as effective as monotherapy for decreasing the risk of clinical progression (66% risk reduction for the combination, 39% for doxazosin, and 34% for finasteride).[4]

UDA analyses also described the use of emerging, minimally invasive surgical therapies for BPH, including laser ablation, transurethral needle ablation, transurethral microwave therapy, high-energy focused ultrasound, and hot water thermotherapy. According to data from the Health care Cost and Use Project, inpatient admissions for certain minimally invasive BPH surgeries (transurethral needle ablation and microwave therapy) increased from 1990 through 2000. It is interesting to note that, although these procedures are typically described as "office-based," at least at the beginning of their adoption curve a portion were being performed as inpatient procedures.

BPH procedures in the ambulatory surgery setting increased concurrently. For instance, population-based incidence rates for minimally invasive surgical therapies increased from 264 per 100,000 in 1998 to 357 per 100,000 in 2000. Concurrent with data supporting effective medical therapy for BPH and the introduction of minimally invasive treatment options, national rates of transurethral resection of the prostate decreased steadily in the 1990s.[2]

Urinary Incontinence in Women

Because women may be reluctant to discuss urinary incontinence (UI) with their physicians or believe it is part of normal aging, using physician office visits to describe the prevalence of UI may substantially underestimate its true burden. Population-based data, in contrast, are derived from surveys of individuals who are not necessarily seeking care, and have greater sensitivity for capturing the true burden of UI among American women.

Analyses of population-based data from the National Health and Nutrition Examination Survey (NHANES) estimated a 38% prevalence of UI among women greater than or equal to 60 years old surveyed from 1999 to 2000. When stratified by frequency of episodes, 13.7% of all women in NHANES reported daily incontinence, whereas an additional 10.3% reported weekly incontinence. The prevalence of daily incontinence increased with age, ranging from 12.2% in all women 60 to 64 years old to 19.4% in those greater than or equal to 85 years old.[5] Women with less than a high school education reported incontinence less often than did those with at least a high school education. Prevalence was higher in non-Hispanic white women (41%) than in non-Hispanic black (20%) or Mexican American (36%) women (**Table 4**). These data are consistent with other large, population-based studies that estimate a higher prevalence of UI in non-Hispanic white women than in other ethnic or racial groups.[6,7] The annual rate of hospitalizations for a primary diagnosis of UI, most of which are presumably for incontinence surgery, remained stable at 51 to 54 per 100,000 between 1994 and 1998. The rate decreased to 44 per 100,000 in 2000, consistent with a shift to ambulatory surgery and hospital outpatient treatment of women with incontinence. The annual hospitalization rate was highest for women between the ages of 65 and 74 years (108 per 100,000) and for women residing in the South and West. Urban dwellers had a higher rate of hospitalizations than did rural dwellers. Hospital stays were longer for older women.[5]

In contrast to the decreasing hospitalization rate for incontinence between 1992 and 2000, outpatient visits for UI more than doubled during this period. Physician visits linked with a UI diagnosis increased from 845 per 100,000 women in 1992 to 1845 per 100,000 in 2000. Similarly, visits for which UI was the primary diagnosis increased from 468 per 100,000 in 1992 to 1107 per 100,000 in 2000.[5] Office visits for incontinence by female Medicare beneficiaries ($\geq$65 years old) increased from 1371 per 100,000 in 1992 to 2937 per 100,000 in 1998. The rate in white women approximately doubled that in African American, Asian American, or Pacific Islander women, and was 50% higher than that in Hispanic women.

Despite its adverse quality of life effects, fewer than half of women with incontinence seek care for this chronic condition.[5] Although only a small fraction of women with UI seek surgical intervention, the number treated surgically is nonetheless substantial and accounts for a considerable proportion of incontinence-related expenditures.[8,9] UDA analyses revealed that among women with commercial health insurance the rate of inpatient hospitalizations for incontinence procedures (as the primary or a secondary procedure) ranged from 123 per 100,000 in 1994 to 114 per 100,000 in 2000. Hospitalizations for incontinence surgeries as the primary procedure decreased from 59 per 100,000 women in 1994 to 33 per 100,000 in 2000. Consistent and substantial geographic variation is also noted in rates of incontinence surgery. For instance, between 1994 and 2000 rates of hospitalization for incontinence-related surgery ranged from 74 to 114 per 100,000 women in the Northeast United States to 217 to 306 per 100,000 in the West.[5]

In 1998, collagen injection, pubovaginal sling, and anterior urethropexy were the most commonly performed surgical procedures for female UI. This pattern reflects increased use of pubovaginal slings among incontinent women from 1995 (621 per 100,000 women) to 1998 (2776 per 100,000). Although still common, the number of anterior urethropexies decreased between 1992 (3941 per 100,000) and 1998 (2364 per 100,000). During the same interval, nationwide use of needle suspension procedures (the so-called "Raz" and "Pereyra" procedures) decreased precipitously.

UDA analyses also captured initial trends toward more frequent ambulatory surgical care for female UI. Among commercially insured women less than or equal to age 65, the rate of ambulatory surgery visits for UI increased from 15 per 100,000 in 1994 to 34 per 100,000 in

Table 1
Burden of selected urologic diseases in America in 2000

	No. Visits to Office-Based Physicians (NAMCS) Plus Hospital Outpatient Clinics (NHAMCS)		No. Visits to Emergency Rooms (NHAMCS)	No. Hospital Stays	Total Expenditures (Million $)[a]
	Primary Diagnosis	Any Diagnosis			
Prostate					
Chronic and acute prostatitis	—	1,841,066	—	—	$84,452,000
Benign prostatic hyperplasia	4,418,425	7,797,781	117,413	105,185	$1099.5
Prostate cancer	3,330,196	—	—	—	$1,295,800,312
Bladder					
Interstitial cystitis, painful bladder syndrome	—	—	—	—	$65,927,937
Urinary incontinence in women	1,159,877[c]	2,130,929	—	46,470	$452.8
Urinary incontinence in men	207,595	353,065	—	1332	$10.3
Bladder cancer	—	—	—	—	—
Lower tract transitional cell cancer	—	832,416	—	—	$1,073,803,094
Upper tract transitional cell cancer	—	—	—	—	$64,309,807
Kidney					
Urolithiasis	1,996,907	2,682,290	617,647	177,496	$2067.4
Kidney cancer	—	279,564	—	—	$401,390,672

Pediatric urologic disorders				
Vesicoureteral reflux	83,791[c]	140,098[b]	—	—	$41,725,663
Undescended testis	148,551	215,482	—	—	—
Hypospadias	—	17,364[c]	—	—	$16,563,330
Ureterocele	—	—	—	—	$16,803,712
Male reproductive health				
Infertility	—	158,413[b]	—	—	$17,046,404
Erectile dysfunction	—	2,904,896	—	—	$327,626,849
Peyronie's disease	—	—	—	—	—
Urethral stricture	—	364,389	—	—	$191,074,350
Testicular cancer	—	14,790	—	—	$21,745,500
Infections				
Urinary tract infections in women	6,860,160	8,966,738	1,311,359	245,879	$2474
Urinary tract infections in men	1,409,963	2,049,232	424,705	121,367	$1027.9

[a] Based on data from National Ambulatory Medical Care Survey (NAMCS), National Hospital Ambulatory Medical Care Survey (NHAMCS), Health care Cost and Use Project (HCUP), and Medical Expenditure Panel Survey (MEPS).
[b] Physician office visits only.
[c] Hospital outpatient visits only.

Table 2
Estimated incremental annual expenditures associated with various urologic diagnoses (per individual)

Diagnosis	Individual Annual Cost ($)[a]
Renal cell cancer	12,155
Bladder cancer	9585
Prostate cancer	7019
Testicular cancer	6236
Urinary incontinence	4498
Urolithiasis	4472
Painful bladder syndrome	4396
Interstitial cystitis	4251
Urinary tract infection in men	2829
Chronic and acute prostatitis	1759
Urinary tract infection in women	1574
Benign prostatic hyperplasia	1536
Erectile dysfunction	1101

[a] Privately insured patients 18–64 years old.

2000. Likewise, the rate of ambulatory surgical center visits by older (≥65 years) Medicare beneficiaries with UI increased from 60 per 100,000 in 1992 to 142 per 100,000 in 1998.[5] During this interval, the increasing use of ambulatory surgery likely reflected the emergence of injectable periurethral bulking agents for female stress incontinence.[10]

Urinary Incontinence in Female Nursing Home Residents

Identification of incontinence at the time of nursing home admission, typically relying on resident medical records, suggests that only 1% to 2% have a diagnosis of incontinence.[11] Clinical studies reveal, however, that a much larger proportion actually has UI at nursing home admission.[12] To

Table 3
National physician office and hospital outpatient visits for benign prostatic hyperplasia or lower urinary tract symptoms

	Count	Rate (95% CI)
1994		
Primary reason	2,899,300	6371 (5495–7248)
Any reason	4,603,426	10,116 (8826–11,406)
1996		
Primary reason	3,658,367	7484 (6294–8675)
Any reason	6,112,287	12,505 (10,856–14,153)
1998		
Primary reason	3,990,359	7754 (6281–9226)
Any reason	6,443,185	12,520 (10,531–14,508)
2000		
Primary reason	4,418,425	8201 (6765–9637)
Any reason	7,797,781	14,473 (12,406–16,540)

Rate per 100,000 based on 1994, 1996, 1998, and 2000 population estimates from Current Population Survey for relevant demographic categories of American male civilian noninstitutionalized population ≥40 years old.
Data from Litwin MS, Saigal CS, editors. Urologic diseases in America. NIH Publication No. 07–5512. Washington: US Department of Health and Human Services, Public Health Service, National Institutes of Health, National Institute of Diabetes and Digestive and Kidney Diseases, US Government Publishing Office; 2007.

Table 4
Prevalence of difficulty controlling bladder in women

	Total No.	No. with Difficulty (%)	No. without Difficulty (%)	No. Refused to Answer or Do Not Know (%)
Totals	23,477,726	8,929,543 (38)	14,449,905 (62)	98,278 (0)
Age at screening				
60–64	5,699,785	2,168,863 (38)	3,530,922 (62)	0
65–69	4,895,878	1,785,380 (36)	3,110,498 (64)	0
70–74	4,505,164	1,683,804 (37)	2,818,651 (63)	2709 (0)
75–79	3,453,472	1,515,900 (44)	1,873,616 (54)	63,956 (2)
80–84	2,981,558	989,003 (33)	1,967,390 (66)	25,165 (1)
85+	1,941,869	786,593 (41)	1,148,828 (59)	6448 (0)
Race and ethnicity				
Non-Hispanic white	18,729,539	7,662,444 (41)	11,041,930 (59)	25,165 (0)
Non-Hispanic black	1,941,269	386,480 (20)	1,554,789 (80)	0
Mexican American	649,003	230,567 (36)	409,279 (63)	9157 (1)
Other Hispanic	1,576,419	468,823 (30)	1,107,596 (70)	0
Other race and ethnicity	581,496	181,229 (31)	336,311 (58)	63,956 (11)
Education				
Less than high school	8,374,762	2,692,649 (32)	5,682,113 (68)	0
High school	7,692,149	3,484,970 (45)	4,207,179 (55)	0
High school or greater	7,212,158	2,725,611 (38)	4,461,382 (62)	25,165 (0)
Refused	103,678	26,313 (25)	13,409 (13)	63,956 (62)
Do not know	87,647	0	85,822 (98)	1825 (2)
Missing	7332	0	0	7332 (100)
Poverty-to-income ratio				
0	111,440	31,876 (29)	79,564 (71)	0
Less than 1	3,145,548	1,116,508 (35)	2,026,331 (64)	2709 (0)
1.00–1.84	5,520,548	2,193,641 (40)	3,326,907 (60)	0
Refused	2,090,410	759,112 (36)	1,331,298 (64)	0
Do not know	1,560,474	741,618 (48)	817,031 (52)	1825 (0)
Missing	1,399,975	548,182 (39)	783,214 (56)	68,579 (5)

Based on question KIQ.040, "In the past 12 months, have you had difficulty controlling your bladder, including leaking small amounts of urine when you cough or sneeze?" (do not include bladder control difficulties during pregnancy or recovery from childbirth).

Data from McConnell JD, Roehrborn CG, Bautista OM, et al. The long-term effect of doxazosin, finasteride, and combination therapy on the clinical progression of benign prostatic hyperplasia. N Engl J Med 2003;349:2387–98.

explore this difference, UDA researchers used data from the National Nursing Home Survey to compare administrative and clinical estimates of the prevalence of incontinence within the same vulnerable population.[13]

Among female nursing home residents with an admitting or current diagnosis of incontinence in their medical records 73.8% to 85.4% was identified by the National Nursing Home Survey as having difficulty controlling urination, and 9.5% to 11.7% had an indwelling urethral catheter (or urinary stoma). Moreover, well over half of those with incontinence required personal assistance and almost one fourth required special equipment when using the toilet.[13] Among the entire population of female nursing home residents (regardless of record-based continence status) 56.3% to 58.6% were reported to have difficulty controlling urination. This rate was stable between 1995 and 1999. Fully 56.6% of these patients required personal assistance and 15.2% required special equipment when using the toilet.

Nursing home residents with incontinence were older than those without incontinence. In 1999, 50.7% of incontinent women were greater than or equal to 85 years old, 31.5% were 75 to 84 years old, and 17.8% were less than or equal to 74 years old (**Table 5**). In contrast, 41.5% of those without incontinence were greater than or equal to 85 years old, 32.2% were 75 to 84 years old, and 26.2% less than or equal to 74 years old. Race and ethnicity did not differ between the incontinent and continent nursing home residents (see **Table 5**).[13]

Compared with existing administrative data, UDA analyses identified a much greater prevalence (58.6%) of urinary control problems among women living in nursing homes. More than half of all female nursing home residents had difficulty controlling urination or needed assistance while using the toilet. The sharp divergence between clinical and administrative data highlights the limitations of using medical records alone to study the epidemiology of UI.

Erectile Dysfunction

According to 2001 to 2002 population-based NHANES data, nearly one in five men experience erectile dysfunction (ED), as defined by self-reports that they are sometimes or never able "to get and keep an erection adequate for satisfactory intercourse."[14] Based on this definition, the prevalence of ED in the United States demonstrates a monotonous increase with advancing age, because more than 75% of men older than 75 meet this self-reported diagnostic criterion (compared with fewer than 10% of men $\leq$40).

In terms of resource use, ED-related health care is increasingly provided in the outpatient setting. For instance, among male Medicare beneficiaries the age-adjusted rate of physician office visits with a primary ED diagnosis more than doubled between 1992 (1609 per 100,000) and 1998 (3387 per 100,000). Similar trends exist for national hospital outpatient visits with ED listed as any diagnosis,[15] and these temporal trends are consistent across age, race and ethnicity, and geographic strata. The rising use of physician office and hospital outpatient visits during this interval likely reflects the concurrent introduction of oral phosphodiesterase inhibitors as first-line ED therapy. Also consistent with this explanation is the corresponding decline in ED-related inpatient surgery rates and expenditures in data from the Health care Cost and Use Project and Medicare.

Among Medicare beneficiaries the subsequent decline (after 1998) in the rate of outpatient visits with ED listed as the primary diagnosis may reflect the management of ED by primary care providers without physiologic testing or diagnostic coding. Patients may also have other conditions as the primary reason for the clinic visit. Illustrating this point, UDA investigators observed that although the rate of male Veterans Affairs patients with ED listed as the primary diagnosis remained virtually constant from 2000 to 2003 (2012 per 100,000 in 2000 versus 1981 per 100,000 in 2003), the number of veterans with ED listed as any diagnosis increased by more than 2000 per 100,000 during this interval (3161 per 100,000 in 2000 versus 5236 per 100,000 in 2003).[15] Likewise, analyses of data from the Veterans Affairs Pharmacy Benefits Management Group demonstrated that the number of veterans receiving prescriptions for specific ED drugs increased ninefold from 1999 to 2003 (681 per 100,000 to 6120 per 100,000).

Before the introduction of pharmacologic therapy, penile implants were the only effective treatment for men with ED; accordingly, implants accounted for most ED-related hospitalizations and expenditures. The annual number of penile implants decreased steadily during the 1990s and 2000s, again coincident with the approval of pharmacologic ED therapies (alprostadil penile injections, alprostadil urethral suppositories, and oral sildenafil in 1994, 1996, and 1998, respectively). The mean annual implant case volume at hospitals that perform at least one implant per year decreased from 22 in 1994 to 16.1 in 2000. Not surprisingly, a corresponding trend for overall inpatient hospital stays was noted. Despite the increasing rates of ED diagnosis, the rate of inpatient hospital stays decreased from 8 per 100,000 in 1994 to 4.7 per 100,000 in 2000. This rate reached a nadir in 1998 (3.8 per 100,000), coincident with the introduction of sildenafil. Notably, admissions for penile implant surgery continue to comprise more than 80% of inpatient stays for men with a primary diagnosis of ED.[15]

Until recently, the burden of disease attributable to ED has been insufficiently quantified among nonwhite men. Fortunately, NHANES data now allow estimation of ED prevalence among racial and ethnic minorities in the United States, including Hispanic men who have been historically understudied (**Table 6**). Notably, the prevalence of ED among Hispanic men younger than 50 is roughly twice that among young non-Hispanic men (12.5% versus 4.9%). The heightened risk among Hispanics persists even after adjustment for known ED risk factors, including diabetes, obesity, and hypertension.[14] Many explanations have been suggested to explain the increased risk for ED among Hispanics.[16,17]

Table 5
Female nursing home residents with admitting or current diagnosis of urinary incontinence

	1995		1997		1999	
	Count	Rate (95% CI)	Count	Rate (95% CI)	Count	Rate (95% CI)
Totals	13,915	1237 (949–1524)	20,679	1789 (1435–2143)	15,979	1366 (1050–1681)
Age						
74 or less	2443	1435 (605–2265)	2408	1334 (610–2058)	2827	1389 (588–2190)
75–84	4159	1131 (662–1601)	9029	2428 (1679–3176)	5668	1540 (972–2107)
85 or more	7313	1245 (848–1644)	9242	1531 (1085–1978)	7685	1254 (823–1685)
Race						
White	13,397	1340 (1022–1558)	17,962	1779 (1403–2155)	15,075	1509 (1148–1869)
Other	518	421 (0–905)	2717	1969 (858–3080)	904	554 (58–1051)

Rate per 100,000 nursing home residents in same demographic stratum.
Data from Wessells H, Joyce GF, Wise M, et al. Erectile dysfunction. J Urol 2007;177:1675–81.

Table 6
NHANES erectile dysfunction question by race and ethnicity

Race and Ethnicity	No. Subjects	% Subjects (95% CI)
White (non-Hispanic)		
Always/almost always able	42,166,116	65.8 (61.2–70.3)
Usually able	9,720,185	15.2 (12.5–17.8)
Sometimes able	7,719,574	12 (10.6–13.5)
Never able	4,513,273	7 (5.0–9.0)
Mexican American		
Always/almost always able	4,254,622	64.2 (59.6–68.8)
Usually able	1,331,461	20.1 (15.3–24.9)
Sometimes able	668,185	10.1 (7.4–12.7)
Never able	374,352	5.6 (3.9–7.4)
African American (non-Hispanic)		
Always/almost always able	5,320,404	61.5 (56.5–66.5)
Usually able	1,930,336	22.3 (19.5–25.1)
Sometimes able	1,092,557	12.6 (9.4–15.9)
Never able	307,653	3.6 (1.3–5.8)
Other Hispanic		
Always/almost always able	3,019,237	63.9 (52.3–75.4)
Usually able	657,696	13.9 (0.6–27.3)
Sometimes able	882,115	18.7 (2.7–34.6)
Never able	166,660	3.5 (0.7–6.4)
Other or multiracial		
Always/almost always able	1,766,502	62.9 (49.8–76.1)
Usually able	727,977	25.9 (12.8–39.1)
Sometimes able	289,029	10.3 (3.3–17.3)
Never able	23,673	0.8 (0–2.7)

Based on the question, "How would you describe your ability to get and keep an erection adequate for satisfactory intercourse?" Percentages may not total 100 because of rounding.
Data from Low WY, Wong YL, Zulkifli SN, et al. Malaysian cultural differences in knowledge, attitudes and practices related to erectile dysfunction: focus group discussions. Int J Impot Res 2002;14:440–5.

UROLOGIC CANCERS
Prostate Cancer

Prostate cancer and its treatments are costly and significantly impact quantity and quality of life. Accordingly, recent UDA analyses quantified trends in disease incidence, presentation, and survival, and examined relevant patterns of health care resource use.

Data from the National Cancer Institute's Surveillance, Epidemiology, and End Results (SEER) program demonstrate that prostate cancer incidence rates peaked in 1992 at 237 per 100,000 (age adjusted, all races and ages); declined steeply until 1995; and then increased at approximately 1.7% per year through 2000. In 2000, 2001, and 2002 the annual age-adjusted incidence rates were 180, 181, and 176 per 100,000, respectively.

Most authorities agree that these results reflect the introduction and proliferation of prostate-specific antigen screening, which began in the late 1980s and early 1990s.

Stage at diagnosis among men with incident prostate cancer has also shifted dramatically during the last 20 years. From 1973 to 1979 and 1985 to 1989, 73% of prostate cancer diagnoses were localized or regional. In contrast, during 1995 and 2001, 91% of diagnoses were localized or regional. Across the same three intervals the percentage with distant disease at diagnosis decreased from 20% to 16% to 5%, respectively.[18]

Finally, survival rates have evolved during the last several decades. For instance, in 1973, 63% and 55% of white and black men, respectively, diagnosed with prostate cancer survived 5 years.

By 1981, the corresponding survival rates had increased to approximately 75% and 65%, respectively, for white and African American men, and for 1995 to 2000, 5-year survival improved again to 100% and 96%, respectively, for white and African American men. Nearly all men now diagnosed with local or regional prostate cancer can expect to survive at least 5 (and usually many more) years after diagnosis.[18]

With respect to resource use, estimates from Medicare suggest that in 1992 almost 86,000 men greater than or equal to 65 years old were hospitalized with a primary diagnosis of prostate cancer. In contrast, fewer than 36,000 men in this demographic group had prostate cancer–related hospitalizations in 2001. The age-adjusted rate of inpatient stays declined from 729 to 309 per 100,000 between 1992 and 2001. Rates of inpatient hospitalization for African Americans exceeded those for whites at all time points, likely reflecting the increasing incidence of the disease in this racial group.[18]

Geographic variations in hospitalization rates exist among Medicare beneficiaries with prostate cancer. Although inpatient hospitalizations decreased for all geographic regions between 1992 and 2001, the most precipitous decline occurred in the Western and Northeastern United States. An explanation for this observed trend is corresponding variability in screening and treatment practices during this time. Notably, from 1994 through 2000 hospitalization rates for prostate cancer in rural regions were less than half the rates in urban areas.

The observed changes in inpatient prostate cancer care are related, at least in part, to radical prostatectomy use rates. Hospitalization rates for radical prostatectomy remained stable between 1994 and 1996 at 127 per 100,000 in men older than 40 years before decreasing to 99 per 100,000 in 1998 and then rising again to 108 per 100,000 in 2000. During this period, radical prostatectomy rates increased among younger men (40–54 years) and declined among men greater than or equal to 65 years.[18]

Most prostate cancer survivors receive a significant portion of their care as outpatients. NAMCS data indicate that the annual age-adjusted rate of physician office visits for prostate cancer in 1992 to 2000 was 5001 per 100,000 American men older than 40 years (**Table 7**). During this period, men 75 to 84 years old had the highest rate of office visits (112,069 per 100,000) compared with men 65 to 74 years old (54,445 per 100,000) and those 40 to 64 years old (5930 per 100,000). Older patients are less likely to undergo aggressive therapy for localized disease and more likely to elect conservative management. They may also be more likely to have regular visits for therapeutic hormonal injections, consequently increasing their use of outpatient care.[18]

Bladder Cancer

Bladder cancer represents the fourth most common cancer among Americans.[19] **Table 8** presents the estimated number of incident cases annually by age and year. Overall survival among patients with bladder cancer improved progressively during the last four decades, and currently 5-year survival is estimated at 82% for all stages combined.

During the last decade, the frequency of inpatient hospitalizations for bladder cancer has decreased in Medicare and non-Medicare populations. The rate of inpatient hospitalization for a bladder cancer diagnosis was highest among older patients (80–89 years) and those living in the Northeast. The rate of inpatient hospitalization was also higher in urban than in rural care settings.[20]

Contrasting with this declining use of inpatient care, outpatient visits and ambulatory surgical interventions among patients with bladder cancer have increased. Nationwide, patients of all ages with bladder cancer made 764,267 visits to physicians' offices in 2000, and Medicare beneficiaries alone made 368,200 office visits in 2001. Most of these visits (68%) were to urologists. The overall rate of ambulatory surgery visits by Medicare patients increased globally and among individual race and ethnicity strata. Bladder cancer–related hospital outpatient visits among Medicare beneficiaries increased from 1992 to 1995 before declining.[20]

Patients with SEER stage I (superficial) tumors are responsible for the largest proportion of office visits within the first 12 months following a bladder cancer diagnosis. Significantly, however, visit rates increase in parallel with disease stage.[20] Among patients with a bladder cancer–related office visit within 12 months of diagnosis 92%, 8%, and 18% saw a urologist, medical oncologist, or internist, respectively. The proportion of patients visiting a medical oncologist increased with higher disease stage. Only 36% of patients with SEER stage IV (distant) disease, however, had documented medical oncology visits. Even if it is assumed that visits to internists and physicians of unlisted specialty represent medical oncologist visits, a substantial fraction of patients with SEER stages III (regional) and IV disease did not consult with a physician capable of administering systemic chemotherapy.

Table 7
Physician office visits for prostate cancer listed as primary diagnosis, 1992–2000

	Count	5-y Rate (95% CI)[a]	Average Annualized Rate Per Year	5-y Age-Adjusted Rate[b]
Totals[c]	12,236,564	25,004 (22,810–27,198)	5001	25,034
Age				
40–64	2,118,240	5930 (4647–7212)	1186	—
65–74	4,399,702	54,445 (46,664–62,226)	10,889	—
75–84	4,739,092	112,069 (95,718–128,421)	22,414	—
85+	979,530	108,031 (79,820–136,242)	21,606	—
Race and ethnicity				
White	10,498,163	26,644 (24,119–29,170)	5329	25,313
Other	1,738,401	18,227 (14,001–22,452)	3645	23,366
Region				
Midwest	2,906,931	25,262 (20,840–29,683)	5052	25,086
Northeast	3,718,177	37,425 (31,362–43,488)	7485	36,556
South	3,187,693	18,669 (15,599–21,740)	3734	18,435
West	2,423,763	23,256 (18,398–28,114)	4651	24,738
Metropolitan statistical area (MSA)				
MSA	10,498,173	28,760 (25,998–31,522)	5752	28,935
Non-MSA	1,738,391	13,979 (11,014–16,943)	2796	13,835

[a] Rate per 100,000 is based on 1992, 1994, 1996, 1998, and 2000 population estimates from Current Population Survey and Utilities, Unicon Research Corporation, for relevant demographic categories of United States male civilian noninstitutionalized population.
[b] Grouped years age adjusted to the US Census derived age distribution of the midpoint of years; individual years age adjusted to the US Census derived age distribution of the year under analysis.
[c] Includes persons of missing or unavailable race and ethnicity, and missing MSA.
Data from Konety BR, Joyce GF, Wise M. Bladder and upper tract urothelial cancer. J Urol 2007;177:1636–45.

Not surprisingly, most patients undergo transurethral resection following the initial diagnosis of bladder cancer. The average annualized rate of transurethral resection of bladder tumor in Medicare patients with a bladder cancer diagnosis is 51% and is generally consistent across genders, geographic regions, and racial and ethnic groups. The annualized rate of transurethral resection of bladder tumor does vary by age, ranging from 46% among 65- to 69-year-old Medicare beneficiaries to 60% among 90 to 94 year olds.[20]

Cystectomy rates in patients with newly diagnosed bladder cancer remained generally stable (67–91 per 1000 per year) from 1990 to 1999. The cystectomy rate is age-sensitive, however, with less-frequent use of radical surgery among patients older than age 80. According to SEER data, the highest rates of radical surgery are among patients

Table 8
Estimated new bladder cancer cases in the United States

	Total No. (%)	No. Male (%)	No. Female (%)
1996	52,900 (3.9)	38,300 (5)	14,600 (2.5)
1998	54,400 (4.4)	39,500 (6.3)	14,900 (2.5)
2000	53,200 (4.4)	38,300 (6.2)	14,900 (2.5)
2002	56,500 (4.4)	41,500 (6.5)	15,000 (2.3)
2004	60,240 (4.4)	44,640 (6.4)	15,600 (2.3)

Data from Cancer Statistics, American Cancer Society Surveillance Research.

with stages III and IV cancers.[20] This finding reflects the preferential use of pathologic (rather than clinical) stage in SEER registry data.

Despite evidence supporting advantageous outcomes among patients undergoing continent urinary diversion at the time of radical cystectomy, UDA analyses of Medicare beneficiaries did not identify an appreciable increase in the use of continent reconstructive procedures during the last decade. The likelihood of receiving a continent diversion seems to be inversely associated with age, African American race, and burden of comorbidity, and directly associated with male gender, higher education level, and more recent year of surgery. Moreover, provider level factors are important determinants of the selection of reconstructive technique. Specifically, treatment at academic and National Cancer Institute–designated cancer centers and by high-volume providers is associated with more frequent use of continent reconstruction (**Table 9**).[21]

PEDIATRIC UROLOGIC CONDITIONS
Hypospadias

Hypospadias is a common congenital anomaly cared for by pediatric and general urologists in the United States. Historical estimates suggest that hypospadias is present in 0.3% of male newborns,[22] although more recent data suggest an increase in incidence to 0.8%[23] of white and 0.4%[24] of nonwhite male newborns. Moreover, surveillance data from the United States indicate a near doubling of the hypospadias incidence rate from 1968 through 1993, with an overall annual rate of increase of 1.4%. During this period, analyses identified 2.9% and 5.7% annual increases among white and nonwhite male newborns, respectively.[24]

Despite its rising incidence, the annual number of hypospadias-related hospitalizations decreased by 75% between 1994 (2669 hospitalizations, 2.2 per 100,000 children) and 2000 (849 hospitalizations, 0.6 per 100,000 children), with most occurring among children 0 to 2 years old (**Table 10**). Specifically, the likelihood of being hospitalized for hypospadias is 10 times greater for children younger than 3 years than for those 3 to 10 years old.[25] This observation is consistent with the common practice of performing surgical hypospadias repair in younger children, often during the first year of life.

Despite the trend toward early surgical repair, older children are often hospitalized for treatment of hypospadias-related complications rather than primary repair. Alternatively, some cases may represent late referrals of uncorrected hypospadias.

In 2000, the proportion of hospitalizations for hypospadias among children older than 3 years increased to 28%.[25] This paradoxical observation may reflect a broader trend (not captured by an inpatient database) toward ambulatory hypospadias repair in infants.

Although hospitalization may be necessary following surgical intervention, most care for children with hypospadias is delivered in the outpatient setting. For commercially insured boys younger than age 3, the rate of hypospadias-related ambulatory surgery increased 1.5-fold from 1994 (321 per 100,000) to 2002 (468 per 100,000). For the same population, physician office visits for hypospadias increased concurrently from 429 per 100,000 in 1994 to 655 per 100,000 in 2002. According to data from the National Survey of Ambulatory Surgery, more than 39,000 visits to ambulatory surgery centers for hypospadias repair occurred between 1994 and 1996. Two thirds of these were infant visits. Children in the Northeast and Midwest were more likely to have an ambulatory surgery visit for hypospadias repair than those in the South or West.[25]

Undescended Testis

Also known as "cryptorchidism," undescended testis affects 3% of full-term male newborns and is the most common male genital anomaly identified at birth. The evaluation and surgical treatment for undescended testis occur almost exclusively in the outpatient setting. Between 1992 and 2000 there were 611,647 physician office visits (96 per 100,000 in each year) for undescended testis listed as the primary diagnosis, and most patients were younger than 18 years.[25] National Survey of Ambulatory Surgery data indicate a constant annualized rate of undescended testis–related surgeries (ie, orchiopexy) at about 18 per 100,000 in 1994 to 1996. Although rates of orchiopexy are highest among children 0 to 2 years old (the recommended age range for surgical correction), a substantial minority of procedures were performed in children 3 to 10 years old, suggesting a delay in either diagnosis or intervention. Geographic variation was also noted, with higher ambulatory surgery rates in the Northeast and Midwest than in the South and West.[25]

Vesicoureteral Reflux

The overall incidence of vesicoureteral reflux in the pediatric population is estimated to be 10%. The prevalence is often reported, however, and varies by mode of presentation (eg, prenatally or among children with prior urinary tract infection).[26] Accordingly, reflux occurs in 17.2% of children

Table 9
Multivariate analysis of factors associated with continent reconstruction

Characteristic	Odds Ratio (95% CI)
Age (versus 65–69)	
70–74	0.68 (0.54–0.87)
75–79	0.43 (0.33–0.55)
At least 80	0.19 (0.13–0.27)
Male	1.45 (1.15–1.84)
Race and ethnicity (versus white)	
African American	0.43 (0.25–0.76)
Hispanic	0.92 (0.55–1.53)
Other	1.09 (0.66–1.80)
Married (versus not married)	1.13 (0.90–1.41)
Median income (versus ≥$75,000)[a]	
Less than $20,000	0.70 (0.16–3.07)
$20,000–$49,999	1.22 (0.81–1.84)
$50,000–$74,000	1.43 (1.01–2.01)
College educated (versus less than 25%)[a]	
25%–40%	1.14 (0.81–1.61)
At least 40%	1.54 (1.06–2.23)
Charlson score (versus 0)	
1–2	0.97 (0.79–1.19)
3+	0.71 (0.51–0.97)
SEER registry (versus Los Angeles)	
San Francisco	0.38 (0.26–0.56)
Connecticut	0.15 (0.11–0.22)
Detroit	0.16 (0.11–0.24)
Hawaii	0.10 (0.03–0.29)
Iowa	0.11 (0.07–0.17)
New Mexico	0.39 (0.23–0.66)
Seattle	1.22 (0.88–1.68)
Utah	0.22 (0.12–0.40)
Atlanta	1.17 (0.74–1.86)
San Jose	0.74 (0.48–1.13)
Surgery year (versus 1992–1994)	
1995–1997	1.56 (1.23–1.97)
1998–2000	1.98 (1.53–2.54)
Stage at least III (versus I)	0.85 (0.70–1.03)
Lymph nodes negative	1.04 (0.84–1.28)
Hospital type	
Academic	1.43 (1.14–1.81)
National Cancer Institute cancer center	5.50 (4.20–7.22)
High-volume hospital (versus low)	1.49 (1.19–1.86)

[a] Based on median income and percent college educated in subject's ZIP code.
Data from SEER-Medicare.

Table 10
Inpatient hospital stays for hypospadias listed as primary diagnosis in 1997 and 2000

	1997				2000		
	Count[a]	Rate (95% CI)[b]	Age-Adjusted Rate[c]	% All Hospitalizations	Count[a]	Rate (95% CI)[b]	% All Hospitalizations
Total[d]	1889	5.2 (3.6–6.7)	5.1	0.06	1385	3.7 (2.5–5.0)	0.04
Age							
<3	1421	24 (16–31)	—	0.06	993	17 (11–22)	0.04
3–10	385	2.3 (1.6–3.1)	—	0.10	277	1.6 (0.9–2.4)	0.09
11–17	82	0.6 (0.3–0.9)	—	0.02	114	0.8 (0.4–1.1)	0.03
Race and ethnicity[e]							
White	954	4 (2.7–5.4)	4.1	0.07	643	2.8 (1.8–3.7)	0.04
Black	169	3 (1.5–4.5)	3.1	0.04	132	2.3 (1.4–3.3)	0.03
Hispanic	274	—	4.2	0.07	200	—	0.04
Region							
Midwest	149	1.7 (0.9–2.6)	1.6	0.02	140	—	0.02
Northeast	706	10 (5.6–15)	11	0.11	463	7 (3.5–10)	0.08
South	388	—	3.1	0.03	282	2.2 (1.0–3.5)	0.02
West	646	—	7.2	0.08	499	—	0.06
Metropolitan statistical area (MSA)							
Rural	44	—	—	0.01	25	—	0.01
Urban	1845	6.6 (4.6–8.5)	6.3	0.07	1357	4.7 (3.1–6.2)	0.05

No value indicates that it did not meet standard for reliability or precision.
[a] Counts may not total because of rounding.
[b] Rate per 100,000 is based on 1997 population estimates from Current Population Survey and Utilities, Unicon Research Corporation, for relevant demographic categories of United States male civilian noninstitutional population under age 18.
[c] Age adjusted to 2000 US Census.
[d] Persons of other races, missing race and ethnicity, and missing MSA are included in the totals.
[e] Race and ethnicity breakdown not included because of large percent of missing values in 1997.
Data from HCUP Kids' Inpatient Database.

without prior urinary tract infection, in 40% to 70% with a history of urinary tract infection, and in up to 37% with prenatally detected hydronephrosis.[27]

An underlying diagnosis of reflux is more common among boys than girls with prenatal hydronephrosis. In contrast, in the setting of a diagnostic evaluation after urinary tract infection, reflux is more frequently detected among girls. The prevalence of reflux in African American children with urinary tract infection is less than that in white children up to age 10.[28] Once reflux is discovered, however, its grade and chance of spontaneous resolution are similar for girls of both races.[29]

Among children younger than 18, the annual reflux-related inpatient hospitalization rate was stable between 1994 and 2000 at 6.4 to 7 per 100,000 children. This trend was true for girls and boys, with the girl/boy ratio remaining relatively constant at 3:1. Inpatient hospitalizations are more common among white children. Regionally, the rates have been relatively constant.[30]

NAMCS data indicate that during 5 years sampled between 1992 and 2000, 418,954 office visits (32 per 100,000 in each year) specified reflux as the primary diagnosis. The rates of visits to physician offices doubled between 1994 and 2002 from 12 to 26 per 100,000 for commercially insured children and from 43 to 85 per 100,000 for children covered by Medicaid. This difference is unlikely to be explained fully by a greater severity of vesicoureteral reflux among Medicaid participants. Rather, socioeconomic factors may concurrently influence the frequency of office visits and the occurrence of reflux-related complications. Among commercially insured children, the gender ratio of outpatient visits has been constant over time, and little geographic variation in patterns of ambulatory care has been noted. Overall, the rate of reflux-related ambulatory surgery visits by commercially insured children increased from 3.4 per 100,000 in 1998 to 4.8 per 100,000 in 2002. This may reflect increased use of Deflux implantation in lieu of open surgical correction or more repeat Deflux procedures.[30]

SUMMARY

The burden of urologic disease on the American public by any measure is immense. It is shifting and deserves ongoing attention as a topic of clinical investigation, epidemiologic analyses, and health services research. UDA analyses have leveraged existing national data sets to identify opportunities to improve the quality of care and reduce disparities in care. Documenting emerging and evolving trends in epidemiology, practice patterns, resource use, technology diffusion, and costs for urologic disease has broad implications for quality, access to care, and the equitable allocation of scarce resources in terms of medical services and research budgets. The UDA project represents a major step toward accomplishing these goals. Further details on the methods and results, and free, downloadable UDA chapters, are publicly available at www.uda.niddk.nih.gov and www.udaonline.net.

REFERENCES

1. Litwin MS, Saigal CS, editors. Urologic diseases in America. NIH Publication No. 07–5512. Washington, DC: U.S. Department of Health and Human Services, Public Health Service, National Institutes of Health, National Institute of Diabetes and Digestive and Kidney Diseases, U.S. Government Publishing Office; 2007.
2. Wei JT, Calhoun E, Jacobsen SJ. Urologic diseases in America Project: benign prostatic hyperplasia. J Urol 2005;173(4):1256–61.
3. Gee WF, Holtgrewe HL, Blute ML, et al. 1997 American Urological Association Gallup survey: changes in diagnosis and management of prostate cancer and benign prostatic hyperplasia, and other practice trends from 1994 to 1997. J Urol 1998;160(5):1804–7.
4. McConnell JD, Roehrborn CG, Bautista OM, et al. The long-term effect of doxazosin, finasteride, and combination therapy on the clinical progression of benign prostatic hyperplasia. N Engl J Med 2003;349(25):2387–98.
5. Thom DH, Nygaard IE, Calhoun EA. Urologic Diseases in America Project: urinary incontinence in women-national trends in hospitalizations, office visits, treatment and economic impact. J Urol 2005;173(4):1295–301.
6. Nygaard I, Turvey C, Burns TL, et al. Urinary incontinence and depression in middle-aged United States women. Obstet Gynecol 2003;101(1):149–56.
7. Sampselle CM, Harlow SD, Skurnick J, et al. Urinary incontinence predictors and life impact in ethnically diverse perimenopausal women. Obstet Gynecol 2002;100(6):1230–8.
8. Olsen AL, Smith VJ, Bergstrom JO, et al. Epidemiology of surgically managed pelvic organ prolapse and urinary incontinence. Obstet Gynecol 1997;89(4):501–6.
9. Waetjen LE, Subak LL, Shen H, et al. Stress urinary incontinence surgery in the United States. Obstet Gynecol 2003;101(4):671–6.
10. Leach GE, Dmochowski RR, Appell RA, et al. Female stress urinary incontinence clinical guidelines panel summary report on surgical management of female stress urinary incontinence. The American Urological Association. J Urol 1997;158(3 Pt 1):875–80.
11. Nygaard I, Thom D, Calhoun E. Urinary incontinence in women. In: Litwin MS, Saigal CS, editors. Urologic Diseases in America. NIH Publication No. 07-5512. Washington, DC: U.S. Department of Health and Human Services, Public Health Service, National Institutes of Health, National Institute of Diabetes and Digestive and Kidney Diseases, U.S. Government Publishing Office; 2007. p. 157–91.
12. Coward RT, Horne C, Peek CW. Predicting nursing home admissions among incontinent older adults: a comparison of residential differences across six years. Gerontologist 1995;35(6):732–43.
13. Anger JT, Saigal CS, Pace J, et al. True prevalence of urinary incontinence among female nursing home residents. Urology 2006;67(2):281–7.
14. Saigal CS, Wessells H, Pace J, et al. Predictors and prevalence of erectile dysfunction in a racially diverse population. Arch Intern Med 2006;166(2):207–12.
15. Wessells H, Joyce GF, Wise M, et al. Erectile dysfunction. J Urol 2007;177(5):1675–81.
16. Low WY, Wong YL, Zulkifli SN, et al. Malaysian cultural differences in knowledge, attitudes and practices related to erectile dysfunction: focus group discussions. Int J Impot Res 2002;14(6):440–5.
17. Rosas-Vargas H, Coral-Vazquez RM, Tapia R, et al. Glu298Asp endothelial nitric oxide synthase polymorphism is a risk factor for erectile dysfunction in the Mexican Mestizo population. J Androl 2004;25(5):728–32.
18. Penson DF, Chan JM. Prostate cancer. J Urol 2007;177(6):2020–9.
19. Jemal A, Siegel R, Ward E, et al. Cancer statistics 2007. CA Cancer J Clin 2007;57(1):43–66.
20. Konety BR, Joyce GF, Wise M. Bladder and upper tract urothelial cancer. J Urol 2007;177(5):1636–45.
21. Gore JL, Saigal CS, Hanley JM, et al. Variations in reconstruction after radical cystectomy. Cancer 2006;107(4):729–37.
22. Borer JG, Bauer SB, Peters CA, et al. Tubularized incised plate urethroplasty: expanded use in primary and repeat surgery for hypospadias. J Urol 2001;165(2):581–5.

23. Silver RI. What is the etiology of hypospadias? A review of recent research. Del Med J 2000;72(8):343–7.

24. Paulozzi LJ, Erickson JD, Jackson RJ. Hypospadias trends in two US surveillance systems. Pediatrics 1997;100(5):831–4.

25. Pohl HG, Joyce GF, Wise M, et al. Cryptorchidism and hypospadias. J Urol 2007;177(5):1646–51.

26. Sargent MA. What is the normal prevalence of vesicoureteral reflux? Pediatr Radiol 2000;30(9): 587–93.

27. Smellie JM, Normand IC. Clinical features and significance of urinary tract infection in children. Proc R Soc Med 1966;59(5):415–6.

28. Askari A, Belman AB. Vesicoureteral reflux in black girls. J Urol 1982;127(4):747–8.

29. McLorie GA, McKenna PH, Jumper BM, et al. High grade vesicoureteral reflux: analysis of observational therapy. J Urol 1990;144(2 Pt 2):537–40 [discussion: 545].

30. Pohl HG, Joyce GF, Wise M, et al. Vesicoureteral reflux and ureteroceles. J Urol 2007;177(5):1659–66.

Fixing Health Care Before It Fixes Us

Laurence J. Kotlikoff, PhD

KEYWORDS

- Healthcare • Vouchers • Risk adjustment
- Global healthcare budget • Universal health insurance

Our nation faces three interrelated and grave health care crises. First, more than 47 million Americans, including 8 million children, have no health insurance coverage. In 1987, the uninsured population totaled 32 million. In two decades, there has been nearly a 50 percent rise in the number of Americans without health insurance.

Second, Medicare and Medicaid costs threaten to bankrupt the country. Today's elderly are now receiving more than $15,000 per year, on average, from these programs. In 2030, when all 78 million baby boomers are fully retired, the average benefit will exceed $25,000, in today's dollars. This estimate is based on optimistic assumptions about benefit growth. In 2030, the two programs' annual costs will run close to $2 trillion in today's dollars.

These huge pending annual health care costs are largely responsible for the roughly $70 trillion fiscal gap that separates the present values of projected federal expenditures and receipts. This fiscal gap provides the true measure of our nation's indebtedness because it puts all future net fiscal obligations, implicit and explicit, on an equal footing. Seventy trillion dollars is a huge amount of money, even for an economy as large as ours. It goes well beyond anything the nation can afford.

The third health care crisis involves enormous health care obligations facing employers, many of whom are drowning in health care bills and looking for the exit. Since 2000, the share of employees covered by employer plans has fallen by over one tenth – from 66 percent of employees to 59 percent. This decline is occurring, in part, from the closure of employer plans and, in part, from employees opting out of their employer's health care plans when their employers invite them to share in paying for premium increases.

Employer-sponsored retiree health care plans are relics in the making. Many companies are freezing their retiree health plans; others are simply reneging in full or in part on past health care insurance promises. General Motors, for example, just handed over $32 billion in health care obligations to the United Auto Workers to get out from under the close to $47 billion in future health care benefits that it had promised its retirees.

The interconnections between the three crises are first order. Employers are reacting to the high cost of health care by eliminating their health plans. This is swelling the ranks of the uninsured. As the uninsured run out of funds to cover their health care bill, more and more end up on Medicaid. Since 2000, Medicaid enrollments have soared by 35 percent. And, to close the circle, the fee-for-service reimbursement system used by Medicare and, to a lesser extent, by Medicaid has contributed significantly to the overall rise in the price of health care and, consequently, to the health care costs employers now face.

DEMOGRAPHICS AND HEALTH CARE BENEFIT GROWTH—WHO'S GOING BROKE?

The United States, Spain, Japan, Norway, and Germany are some of the countries in deepest trouble, when measured by their fiscal gaps relative to the gross domestic product (GDP). The trouble stems from three sources: growth in government spending on retirement and health care benefits; growth in government purchases of goods and services; and changes in demographics.

Demographic change is already here. In Japan, 18 percent of the population is now 65 years and older. America's oldest baby boomer is now eligible for early social security retirement benefits. The

Department of Economics, Boston University, 270 Bay State Road, Boston, MA 02215, USA
E-mail address: kotlikoff@bu.edu

Urol Clin N Am 36 (2009) 29–36
doi:10.1016/j.ucl.2008.08.011

European and Japanese workforces are already shrinking, and Japan's population growth rate is already negative. Europe's population growth rate will turn negative in just 4 years.

As **Table 1** indicates, the United States is now and will remain significantly younger than Japan and Germany. Canada's elderly population share will be similar to that of the United States for the next three decades, but then Canada will get older than the United States. By midcentury, Canada's oldsters will represent 26.7 percent of the population compared with 21.3 percent in the United States. In time, even China, which is now much younger than is the United States, will be older than the United States. Although the United States will be the young kid on the block, even the United States will look very old. The entire country will be older than current-day Florida. And there will be more than just a large number of oldsters. There will be a lot of old oldsters: people who are 85 years and older. Indeed, in 2050, there will be enough Americans who are 85 years and older to fill up all of New York City, Los Angeles, and Chicago. There will be enough centenarians to fill up all of Washington, D.C.!

Fertility is the major force determining long-run aging. As **Fig. 1** shows, postwar fertility changes have been extraordinary. In1950, the fertility rate in China was 6.22 percent; now. it's about 1.7. In the United States, it was 3.45 percent; now, it's about 2.11. There are also amazing fertility rates in Europe and Russia. Italy's rate is currently 1.2 percent. In Japan, the rate is 1.3 percent. In Russia, it's 1.1 percent. These incredibly low fertility rates presage, of course, major declines in population.

Longevity increases are also playing and will continue to play an important role in the aging process. **Fig. 2** shows dramatic change – past and projected – in life expectancy in the United States, China, Germany, and Japan.

Consider Japanese newborns born in 2050. They will live, on average, to age 88. In 2050, the median age in Japan will be 52. In 1950, the median age in Japan was 22.

Past and projected fertility and longevity changes have important implications for total population sizes. As **Fig. 2** shows, the United State's population will expand by about 100 million people through the middle of the century. This is a projected 33 percent increase compared with the current total.

In Europe, there will be a major depopulation – by roughly 80 million – over the same time period. Russia's and Japan's populations will fall by about 20 percent. If fertility rates don't turn around, by the end of the century, Russia's and Japan's populations will be roughly half of what they are today (**Fig. 3**).

PAYING THE PIPER

These projected demographic changes are fascinating, but what are their fiscal implications? Consider the United States, which now spends over $30,000 per old person on Social Security, Medicare, and Medicaid. Medicare is the old-age health insurance program run by the federal government. Medicaid is the government's health care program for the poor, including poor elderly in nursing homes. Because of the high costs of nursing homes, about 70 percent of total Medicaid expenditures is spent on the elderly.

If $30,000 seems like a lot of money, it is. It's about 80 percent of United States per capita GDP. It's higher than the GDP per capita in about 200 of the world's 231 countries. However, by 2030, when the baby boomers are fully retired, the average benefit level per oldster won't be $30,000; it will be at least $50,000 (measured in today's dollars) and represent more than 100 percent of 2030 per capita United States GDP. The remarkably high levels of oldster benefits, current and projected, are due, in the main, to the growth in the health care component of total Social Security, Medicare, and Medicaid outlays.

The table below details real government health care benefit-level growth in the United States, Japan, Canada, and Germany between 1970 and 2002. In the case of the United States, the real

Table 1
Elderly population shares

Country	2005 (%)	2030 (%)	2050 (%)	2070 (%)
Germany	17.1	26.3	30.5	31.3
Japan	18.0	29.9	36.8	37.7
United States	12.4	19.1	21.3	21.6
Canada	13.0	23.6	26.7	27.1
China	7.6	16.3	23.5	na

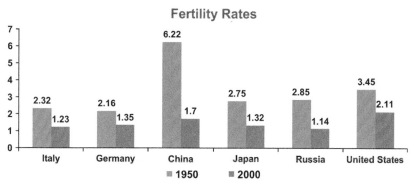

Fig. 1. Fertility rates by country, for the years 1950 and 2000.

growth rate of the benefit level (measured as Medicare and Medicaid expenditures per person at a given age) averaged 4.61 percent per year. In Germany, real benefit-level growth averaged 3.3 percent; in Japan, it averaged 3.6 percent. In the United States, the 1970–2002 health care benefit level growth rate exceeded the corresponding growth rate of per capita GDP by a factor of 2.3. The rate of growth of health care benefit levels in the United States and other countries is clearly unsustainable, but when will it end?

THINGS THAT CAN'T GO ON CAN STOP TOO LATE

The late, great economist Herb Stein was famous for saying, "Things that can't go on will stop." However, what Stein left out was: that things that can't go on can stop too late. Dealing with our current $70 trillion fiscal gap is a Herculean task. Delaying that adjustment will make the adjustment that much harder.

To get a sense of what $70 trillion really means note that closing this gap would require an immediate and permanent doubling of United States payroll taxes, which now represent 15.3 percent of covered wages. Alternatively, one could collect $70 trillion in present value by eliminating all federal discretionary spending for all time. This means no military, no Air Force One, no judicial system, no pay for Congress, and no road construction, for example.

It would be nice were the $70 trillion a figment of an errant academic's dismal imagination. The figure, however, comes not from an academic. Instead, it comes by way of the U.S. Treasury Department; indeed, the $70 trillion figure reflects an update of a 2002 study prepared by then United States government economists, Jagadeesh Gokhale and Kent Smetters, who prepared a fiscal gap analysis at the request of then Treasury Secretary Paul O'Neill (**Table 2**).

How can the United States fiscal gap be so big? When you are projecting paying $50,000, on average, to upwards of 77 million baby boomers, you're talking about spending close to four trillion dollars a year in today's dollars. Yes, the United States economy will be larger when these payments are made to the boomers, but four trillion

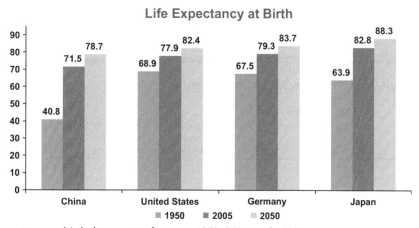

Fig. 2. Life expectancy at birth, by country, for years 1950, 2005, and 2050.

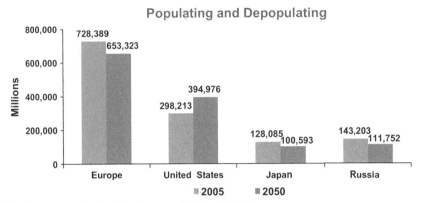

Fig. 3. Population by country/region for the years 2005 and 2050.

dollars a year is still a huge expenditure to be making each and every year.

What's particularly troubling is that the $70 trillion fiscal gap estimate is based on quite optimistic assumptions. The estimate assumes the health care benefit growth rate will be about 3.1 percent rather than the 4.6 percent rate recorded between 1970 and 2002. Unfortunately, there is no reason to expect a decline in the growth rate of the combined Medicare and Medicaid benefit level. Indeed, in the last seven years, this benefit-level growth rate has averaged about 5.6 percent in real terms, not 3.1 percent!

MACROECONOMIC FALLOUT

Any reasonable observer considering the size of the United States fiscal gap must conclude that the United States is, quite literally, facing bankruptcy. Bankruptcy is a strong term. In a business context, bankruptcy means future earnings can't cover future costs as well as current unpaid bills. It also means defaulting on creditors. In a government context, bankruptcy means future receipts that don't cover future expenditures. It also means defaulting on creditors: all those expecting to receive

government health care, pension, welfare, and other benefits as well as all those expecting to be employed by the government. Government bankruptcy also means jacking up tax rates and printing money to "pay" for what the government spends.

No doubt, there are some people who believe that the United States is immune from fiscal meltdown and high inflation, if not hyperinflation. They should think again. Too many countries, big and small, rich and poor, have demonstrated that, sooner or later, fiscal profligacy comes at a very heavy price. Indeed, our current severe contraction is being fueled by a degree of pessimism far beyond anything we've seen in postwar recessions. This loss of confidence in the U.S. economy is surely greatly exacerbated by the public's strong sense that the federal government's long-run fiscal position is unsustainable.

There are increasing signs that Uncle Sam is driving the United States economy over the cliff and that the rest of the world is taking notice. The United States national saving rate is now running below 3 percent. In 1960, it was close to 13 percent. Our incredibly low saving rate has lead to an incredibly high current account deficit, which has led to an incredibly low value of the dollar.

Table 2
1970–2002 Growth in government health care benefit levels

Country	Annual Growth in Expenditure Per Potential Recipient (%)	Annual Growth in Expenditure Per Capital (%)	Annual Growth in GDP Per Capital (%)	Ratio of Column One to Column Three
Germany	3.30	3.62	1.54	2.1
Canada	2.32	3.08	2.04	1.1
Japan	3.57	4.85	2.44	1.5
United States	4.61	5.10	2.01	2.3

Why is the United States saving rate so low? The answer is clear. The counterpart of saving too little is consuming too much. As a share of national income, the federal government is consuming at roughly twice the rate it did a decade ago. But the main explanation for the decline in United States saving is not Uncle Sam's spending. It's the spending – the consumption – of households. The households whose consumption have been rising most rapidly are those of the elderly. Since 1960, average consumption per oldster has roughly doubled relative to average consumption per youngster.

Who is paying for this growth in the consumption of oldsters? The answer, in large part, is Uncle Sam. With Medicare and Medicaid benefits, for example, the vast majority of which go to the elderly. Every year that Uncle Sam allows these benefits to grow much more rapidly than the economy – and this means virtually each of the past 60 years – the government directly expands the consumption of the elderly and, thereby, national saving. Uncle Sam has also been cutting taxes on the elderly, which has also permitted them to consume a lot more.

Uncle Sam's policy of taking ever larger resources from young savers and handing them to old spenders, increasingly in the form of in-kind medical goods and services, is showing up in the level of consumption of the elderly, in the rate of aggregate United States consumption, in the United States national saving, in the country's current account deficit, and in the value of the dollar.

FISCAL GAPS IN OTHER COUNTRIES

Unfortunately, recent fiscal gap analyses are not available from other countries for comparison with the gap in the United States, but the United States may not be alone with respect to long-term fiscal insolvency. This author contends that Spain, Japan, Norway, and Germany are also in very bad long-term shape. However, each of these countries has a health care system directly controlled by its government; each of these countries is in a much better position to stop, on a dime if need be, excessive health care spending.

Consider Canada, for example. It has a state pension system that appears to be in long-run actuarial balance and one of the lowest real health care benefit growth rates in the Organization for Economic Cooperation and Development (OECD). As **Table 2** shows, real government health care benefit levels are growing in Canada at essentially the same rate as per capita GDP. On the other hand, because of the demographics, total expenditures per capita on health care in Canada have grown more rapidly than has per

capita GDP. Canada also has a health care spending problem, but it is largely driven by demographics and it's a problem, not a crisis.

THE UNITED STATES HEALTH CARE CRISIS

Much of the recent growth in United States government health care benefit levels has to do with the number of people who are collecting benefits at a given age, but the benefit level referenced here is not benefits per Medicare and Medicaid recipient at a given age. Rather, it is the benefits per person at a given age. Growth in government health care benefits per person at a given age reflects both the growth in benefits per recipient at that age and the growth in the age-specific participation rate.

There has been an enormous increase in age-specific Medicaid participation rates since 2000. Indeed, as indicated, overall Medicaid participation has increased by over one third since President Bush took office. Part of this expansion of Medicaid reflects the recent enrollment of millions of otherwise uninsured children via what is called the State Child Health Insurance Program (SCHIP) program.

The health care crisis is not simply a problem on its own. It's a problem that greatly compounds the United States fiscal crisis. President-elect Obama has been promising to provide major health care insurance subsidies to millions of uninsured Americans while simultaneously expanding Medicaid and also leaving Medicare unreformed. The United States desperately needs universal health insurance, but it needs to be implemented in a way that doesn't put the final nail in the United States fiscal coffin.

POLITICAL "SOLUTIONS"

The major Democratic presidential candidates are advocating policies that address only one of our three health care problems: the 47 million uninsured. Their method of covering the uninsured could exacerbate the other two crises. Their plan is to place all 47 million uninsured people in a huge pool. Low-income uninsured households would receive an income-related subsidy to buy insurance. Middle- and high-income households would not. Insurers providing coverage to anyone in the pool would be required to cover everyone who applies. Under some proposals, the uninsured would be forced to either buy a policy or face a tax or some other form of punishment.

The plans also envision giving the uninsured the option to receive coverage from a new Medicare-type government entity, which, presumably, would provide fee-for-service payments to providers in a manner analogous to the workings of Medicare Part A and Part B. This new Medicare program, which this author will call Part E, is envisioned, presumably, to ensure that middle class uninsured, with incomes too high to be subsidized, will still be able to buy a policy at a reasonable price.

The subsidization of the low-income uninsureds' purchase of insurance and the creation of Medicare Part E represents the establishment of another major government health care program at a time when the existing ones are out of control, with respect to their costs, and are, on their own, fully capable of driving the nation broke.

THE GREAT UNRAVELING

Traditional employer-based health insurance is already unraveling, but the introduction of major subsidies to the low-income uninsured and the establishment of Medicare Part E could dramatically accelerate this process. Employers could well tell their low-income workers: "The government has established a new health insurance system for which you are eligible. If you opt out of our plan and join the government's, you can receive a subsidy."

This invitation by employers to their employees to, in effect, "get lost" when it comes to their health care, is, after all, what has been happening for years with respect to employer-provided health care for retirees. Employers have realized that duplicating Medicare's coverage makes no sense and that the cheaper way to go is to compensate their workers in other forms and arrange to have their workers go onto Medicare when they retire.

Even high-income workers might be induced by their employers or, indeed, compelled, if employers cancels their health plans, to switch to "uninsureds' insurance." The government will be under great pressure to ensure that premiums charged by participating "uninsureds'" insurers and by Medicare part E are affordable by the middle class members who won't qualify for subsidization. This is particularly the case if the government chooses to force the uninsured middle class, at pain of penalty, to buy coverage. If the government is going to force the public to buy something, it has to be something good and it has to be something affordable. If it is good coverage and affordable for the uninsured middle class, it will also be good coverage and affordable for the middle class who are currently covered by employer plans. Yes, employers who don't provide their own plans will be forced to pay a tax to help pay for their workers, but if that tax is not too high, it may well behoove them to close their plans or encourage many of their workers to opt out of their plans. Massachusetts' health care reform provides an object lesson. The plan sets up a new, subsidized system for the uninsured and compels the uninsured to enroll. It also forces employers to pay a tax per employee if they don't cover the worker under a plan of their own. Costs of the reform have skyrocketed, even though the reform has just begun. Enrollment in the plan is twice the amount originally forecast, according to "Subsidized Care Plan's Cost to Double," *The Boston Globe*, February 3, 2008. The tax being charged employers is incredibly low: less than $300 per year per employee. Massachusetts had planned for the federal government to pick up half of the tab of the program, but that seems highly unlikely. Indeed, Massachusetts' as well as other states' planned major expansions of SCHIP, which insures children under Medicaid, have been thwarted by repeated presidential veto.

IS UNIVERSAL HEALTH CARE AFFORDABLE?

Our country's fiscal gap is so massive that an immediate and permanent doubling of the 15.3 percent employer plus employee payroll tax would be required to close it. That represents a huge potential tax hike and one that would very badly undermine work incentives. Other taxes could, of course, be raised to close the fiscal gap, but such adjustments would be no less painful.

Given our massive fiscal gap, worsening Medicaid's finances and letting Medicare's further hemorrhage, which is precisely what our politicians are promising, will leave no money for anything else, let alone massive government subsidies to assist tens of millions of low-income uninsured households to buy insurance. Rather than help employers exit the health insurance business, these schemes permanently trap all employers in it. Worse yet, they may suggest to employers that they should dump their plans and simply pay the insurance tax for all their workers, lest the government pass a law that compels them to indefinitely maintain their current, very expensive plans.

With regard to forcing the uninsured poor to pay for their own coverage, "good luck". There is no way to force someone who is poor to buy health insurance, resulting in an army of uninsured when all is said and done. What's needed is a universal health care plan that provides a single fix for all three of our crises. This author calls the solution the "Medical Security System." The 10-point plan is simple and is described here.

THE MEDICAL SECURITY SYSTEM

1. The plan provides universal coverage. The Medical Security System would replace our current Medicare, Medicaid and employer-based health care systems.
2. The plan provides each American each year with a health insurance voucher.
3. Those with higher expected health care costs receive bigger vouchers; indeed, vouchers would be proportional to expected health care costs. (There would be with some additional adjustment to the size of the voucher for those with high upside-cost risk.)
4. Each year participants use their voucher to purchase a basic health plan.
5. Participants can change their health plans annually.
6. The basic policy will cover prescription drugs, home health care, and nursing home care.
7. An independent, government-appointed panel of doctors, hospital administrators, insurance executives, patient representatives, and government officials define the basic policy.
8. Each plan must cover the basic policy and accept any and all Americans who wish to join the plan (ie, buy the policy with their voucher).
9. Health plans are free, within limits set by the panel, to compete for participants via co-payment rates and deductibles, as well as incentives to exercise, reduce weight, stop smoking, and otherwise improve health.
10. The government fixes its total annual voucher budget as a fixed share of GDP so that the nation can't go broke due to health care expenditures.

DISCUSSION

The best part of the plan is that it requires very little new financing. Add up everything federal and state government will shortly be shelling out on health care both directly and indirectly via tax breaks; throw in some significant administrative savings; and the sum is roughly 90% of the money needed to pay for the Medical Security System.

In addition to resolving three terrible problems, the plan is highly progressive. It eliminates huge tax breaks to the rich and provides vouchers based on medical condition. Because the poor are, on average, in worse health than the rich, they will, on average, receive larger vouchers than the rich, at a given age.

Finally, The Health Care Fix preserves and, in fact, would greatly strengthen our competitive health care industry. The plan institutes universal health insurance, not universal health care per se, although universal health care is the end result. The distinction is important.

What is being proposed here is not a government-run health care system. It is a plan for the government to redirect its current expenditures to a new system that is efficient, equitable and highly competitive — and one that won't drive our nation broke.

Each insurance company would make a small profit on the vouchers. There would still be private provision (ie, private competition by the hospitals and the doctors), but there would also be socialized finance of health insurance. This isn't universal health care per se; it's universal health insurance. The health care would continue to come from the private sector.

HOW THE MEDICAL SECURITY SYSTEM WOULD WORK

In October of each year, each American would receive a voucher with the size of the voucher depending on the person's objective health conditions. If Mr. Jones has cancer, he gets a big voucher. If he is perfectly healthy, he gets a small voucher. Each person would be individually risk-adjusted to determine the size of the voucher. Each person would spend the voucher, by January 1st, on a health pan, which would cover him or her for the year.

The government would transmit the amount of money on the voucher to the insurance company chosen. At that point, the insurance company is on the line to pay for all health care costs covered by the basic plan.

Households would be free to purchase supplemental insurance from their basic plan provider to cover health care expenditures not covered under the basic plan. Such excluded costs include paying for a private hospital room, paying for the use of new equipment and procedures not covered by the basic plan, and paying for prescription drugs not covered by the basic plan.

Each person's medical tests, scans, x-rays, prescriptions, and objective diagnoses would be entered electronically into a government health care database creating an electronic medical record (EMR) for each American. The EMRs would be used to risk-adjust each person each year. And this objective risk adjustment would, in turn, be used to determine the size of the person's voucher.

The risk adjustment would take into account regional costs, but one could not garner a larger voucher by incurring more health care expenses on one's behalf. One's health care expenses, per se, would have no impact on the size voucher one receives. Instead, one's voucher will depend solely on objective test results and other data concerning one's health status.

Because insurers will be compensated for taking on people with pre-existing conditions, they will stop trying to cherry pick the market and start focusing on providing the best care and insurance arrangements for their clients, including the sickest among them. In economic terms, the Medical Security System solves the adverse selection problem that plagues the private health insurance market.

However, adverse selection is not the only problem undermining private insurance and private care. This new plan also calls for medical malpractice legislation, which would limit defensive medicine and permit insurance companies, subject to appeal to the panel, the right to deny coverage for care not approved by the panel as part of the basic plan.

The Medical Security System also acknowledges that we can not perfectly risk adjust, although one can do a much better job than is being done today, for example, in Medicare Part C. To deal with imperfections in risk adjustment, the government would establish a re-insurance system that pools risks across insurance companies for covering patients who turn out to be extremely expensive.

The Medical Security System would naturally encourage insurance companies to join with providers in forming Accountable Care Organizations (ACOs) or Physician-Hospital Organizations (PHOs). Kaiser-Permanente is an example of such an organization. Insurance companies could offer either "at risk" contracts with organizations or provide administrative services for ACOs/PHOs large enough to self-insure.

Under the Medical Security System the government would also: a) provide incentives for providers to provide coordinated care and develop team approaches to health care; b) intervene to address local medical monopolies that attempt to charge prices far above national standards; c) use the EMRs inputs and outcomes data to engage in comparative effectiveness/resource-use efficiency research; d) disseminate to the public information on costs, quality, and treatment modalities; e) use EMRs to help the private sector achieve the numerous and important specific health improvements and cost savings that George Halvorson outlines in his recent book *Healthcare Reform Now!*[1]; f) set up an Internet system for the public to use to spend their voucher (ie, to choose particular health plans); and g) organize default insurance plans for those who fail to select an insurance plan by January first of each year.

SUMMARY

The current American health care system is beyond repair. It needs to be replaced in its entirety with a new system that provides every American with first-rate, first-tier medicine and that doesn't drive our nation broke. The Medical Security System proposed here may sound radical, but what's truly radical is maintaining the "suicidal" status quo.

The Medical Security System should appeal to both Democrats and Republicans. For Democrats, the plan offers universal health insurance, publicly financed, and provided on a progressive basis. For Republicans, the plan maintains our private and competitive health care provider system as well as our system of private health care insurance. It also permits insurance companies to innovate and to give people incentives to: a) neither under- or overuse the health care system; and b) to improve their health. Additionally, this new plan would make it clear to all Americans, in sending them an explicit voucher, that they are, at the margin, buying their health care and that they need to spend their voucher in a way that provides them the most value for the money.

The Medical Security System should also appeal to the uninsured, those in Medicaid and Medicare, and even those now covered by employer plans. The uninsured will obviously benefit from a system in which their basic health care is as good as everyone else's. Medicaid participants will benefit from being in a system that no longer cuts off their insurance coverage if they earn or save too much money. Medicare participants will realize that their future health care benefits are no longer jeopardized by a system that is going broke and increasingly leading their doctors to say, "I don't take Medicare." Finally, those who are covered by their employers' plans will realize that they too are uninsured under the current system because they too can end up, at any time, among the ranks of the uninsured or find they need to cover the health care costs of their uninsured friends and relatives.

No system is perfect and the Medical Security System no doubt has its shortcomings, but piecemeal United States health care reform, of the kind now being discussed, is a prescription for putting both our health care and our economy at extremely grave risk.

REFERENCE

1. Halvorson G. Healthcare Reform Now! New York: Jossey-Bass; 2007.

Performance Measurement, Public Reporting, and Pay-for-Performance

Kim F. Rhoads, MD, MPH[a,b], Badrinath M. Konety, MD, MBA[c,d],
R. Adams Dudley, MD, MBA[b,e],*

KEYWORDS

- Performance measurement • Public reporting
- Pay-for-performance
- Health care quality improvement • Urology

The use of incentives to improve quality of care is spreading rapidly across the health care system. In some cases, this involves public reporting (PR) (a reputational incentive to do well); in others it involves direct financial incentives such as pay-for-performance (PFP). Both of these strategies are central to Medicare's new value-driven health care initiative.[1] From an historical standpoint, the use of incentives to improve quality is not entirely new. PR, in particular, started in the mid-1980s and has grown slowly. By 2007, six state governments had instituted PR for surgical mortality rates (most often for cardiac surgery), and ten states issued hospital report cards that addressed topics ranging from surgical complications and mortality to compliance with preventive care guidelines in nonsurgical patients. The impact of PR over the past two decades has been limited, however. Signs of underuse of publicly reported data appeared in the literature in the late 1990s. A cohesive body of evidence suggests that third-party payers, patients, and referring physicians rarely used the data in early public reports to make clinical decisions.[2–4] Most patients were completely unaware of the existence of such information.[4]

More recently, economic solutions to the nation's health care crisis have been put forth. Increasingly, the effort to improve health care quality is linked to efforts to maximize the value received for each dollar spent on health care and the goal of assigning accountability for the quality of care to hospitals and individual practitioners. These principles have been combined into PFP programs, such as California's Integrated Health care Association (IHA) and Massachusetts Health Quality Partners. Both are nonprofit collaborative groups in which physicians interact with insurance companies, employers, and consumers to select quality measures. In IHA and Massachusetts Health Quality Partners, the major health plan partners have used the selected quality measures as the basis for PFP to physicians.

PR and PFP are emerging as the dominant models of incentive-based programs designed to

Dr. Dudley's work on this article was funded by a Robert Wood Johnson Foundation Investigator Award in Health Policy.

[a] Department of Surgery, Stanford University, 300 Pasteur Drive, H3680, Stanford, CA 94305, USA
[b] Institute for Health Policy Studies, Box 0936, University of California, 3333 California Street, Suite 265, San Francisco, CA 94118, USA
[c] Department of Urology, University of California, Box 1695, San Francisco, CA 94143-1695, USA
[d] Department of Epidemiology and Biostatistics, University of California, 185 Berry Street, Lobby 5, Suite 5700, Box 0560, San Francisco, CA 94107, USA
[e] Division of Pulmonary and Critical Care Medicine, 400 Parnassus Avenue #5, University of California, San Francisco, CA 94143, USA
* Corresponding author. Institute for Health Policy Studies, University of California, San Francisco, Box 0936, 3333 California Street, Suite 265, San Francisco, CA 94118.
E-mail address: adams.dudley@ucsf.edu (R.A. Dudley).

motivate hospitals and health care providers to improve quality and efficiency. The main incentives associated with PR for hospitals and providers include improved reputation and the potential to increase market share. Although the exact measures vary among PR and PFP programs, most share a common goal of improving the quality of care delivered, motivated by economic benefits (eg, market share, direct financial reward) or penalties (eg, loss of reputation, loss of reimbursement).

CURRENT PUBLIC REPORTING PROGRAMS

Given the rapid spread of PR initiatives, it is beyond the scope of this srticle to describe the full range of programs currently underway around the nation. To give a sense of what some providers face, however, we outline the ongoing PR activities operating in a single state, California. Although California may have more initiatives than some other states, the programs there likely reflect the direction the nation is heading and can help providers everywhere understand what they may face at some point in the future.

PR programs in California were originally initiated by the state government through its Office of Statewide Health Planning and Development, which first started reporting publicly hospital-specific, risk-adjusted mortality rates for various conditions (myocardial infarction was the first) in the 1990s. Since then, other state regulatory agencies, employer groups, multi-stakeholder collaboratives, and even providers themselves have adopted PR. For example, efforts to create incentive-based quality improvement programs for California physicians have been led by the IHA. The IHA is a multi-stakeholder coalition whose membership includes major health plans, physician groups, and hospital systems, which work together with academic, consumer, purchaser, pharmaceutical, and health care technology representatives. Among the group's principal projects are performance assessment and PR programs. **Table 1** summarizes current PR projects supported by IHA members and other major PR activities ongoing in California.[5] California providers are also subject to national PR initiatives such as PR about hospital performance by the Joint Commission on Accreditation of Health care Organization (JCAHO).

CURRENT PAY-FOR-PERFORMANCE PROGRAMS

The Leapfrog Group, a coalition of large employers that seeks to improve the quality of health care and collectively covers approximately 40 million beneficiaries, maintains a compendium of PFP programs on its Web site.[6] In 2006, the compendium included more than 100 PFP programs nationwide. In the United States, more than half the health maintenance organizations in the private sector, a group that collectively has more than 80% of health maintenance organization enrollees, have initiated such programs.

Although still in early phases, the US Congress recently mandated the Center for Medicare and Medicaid Services (CMS) to develop a plan to introduce PFP programs into Medicare. To address this, CMS has engaged in several demonstration projects. In the Premier hospital quality improvement demonstration project, CMS has partnered with Premier, a national hospital performance improvement alliance based in North Carolina whose participants comprise 1700 not-for-profit hospitals and health systems with the core purpose "to improve the health of communities."[7] CMS and Premier have adopted a set of performance indicators based on validated measures adapted from the American Hospital Association, the National Quality Forum, JCAHO, the Leapfrog Group and the federal Agency for Healthcare Research and Quality.

Table 2 lists the process and outcome measures being used in the CMS Premier demonstration project,[8] such as measures for patients with myocardial infarction, heart failure, pneumonia, coronary artery bypass graft, hip, and knee replacement surgeries. CMS calculates annual composite quality scores for each clinical condition for each hospital by combining performance scores for each individual measure within the clinical area. Hospitals in the top 10% for a given clinical area receive a bonus of 2% of their Medicare payments for the measured condition, whereas hospitals in the second decile are paid a 1% bonus. In the third year of the demonstration project, hospitals that fail to score above the levels that represented the thresholds for ninth and tenth deciles of performance in the first year of the program suffer 1% and 2% lower diagnostic related group (DRG) payments, respectively. By using the thresholds defined in the first year of the program for the penalty portion of the demonstration, CMS gave all hospitals the opportunity to improve above a known target and avoid creating a situation in which 20% of participating hospitals would have been guaranteed a penalty (which would have happened if they had used current year performance).

ASSESSING QUALITY OF CARE: KEY CONCEPTS

Whether PR and PFP improve quality of care is not yet certain. Most of what we know about how people respond to incentive-based programs has

Table 1
A selection of public reporting projects active in California as of December 2006[5]

Project Title/Sponsor	Start Date	Program/Project Description	Incentive
California Hospital Assessment and Reporting Taskforce (CHART)/California Health care Foundation, California health plans	2005	System of California hospital report cards, with results available on line at www.calhospitalcompare.org	Reputation, market share
KP Public Reporting/ Kaiser Permanente Northern California Region	2006	Creates a report cared for hospitals and medical offices for publication on Kaiser Permanente Web site	Reputation
Leapfrog California Patient Safety Initiative/Pacific Business Group on Health	2002	Program to reduce preventable medical errors in hospitals and create consumer choice tools; results to be published online on various consumer health sites	Reputation, market share
Medi-Cal Auto Assignment Project/ California Health and Human Services Agency	2005	Program compares performance of health plans within same geographic area on five HEDIS measures with public reporting on performance	Market share
Patient Assessment Survey/Pacific Business Group on Health	2001	Annual survey measuring patient experience at the physician group level; publicly reported data intended for use by consumers and health plans via PFP mechanism	Reputation, market share
Pay for Performance Program/IHA	2002	The goal is to reward physician groups for performance in clinical care and patient experience based on public reporting	Reputation, market share

emerged from studies conducted in other fields, such as economics, psychology, and organizational behavior. The theoretic frameworks developed within these fields are not necessarily directly applicable to health care,[9] partly because of the complex web of relationships among physicians, patients, third-party payers, and purchasers of health insurance, which makes it difficult to study, let alone confidently identify, the key factors influencing provider and consumer responses to PR or PFP. We do know that although PR and PFP may create incentives, they do so in a milieu rich with myriad existing financial incentives. On one hand, traditional fee-for-service insurance creates incentives to provide more services, while on the other hand, capitation creates incentives to

Table 2
The Centers for Medicare and Medicaid Services/premier hospital quality incentive demonstration project clinical conditions and measures for reporting[8]

CMS Premier Focus Area	Process Measures	Outcome Measures
Acute myocardial infarction	Aspirin at arrival Aspirin at discharge Angiotensin converting enzyme inhibitor (ACEI) for left ventricular systolic dysfunction Smoking cessation advice/ counseling Beta-blocker at discharge Beta-blocker at arrival Thrombolytic therapy within 30 minutes of hospital arrival Percutaneous coronary interventions (PCI) received within 120 minutes of hospital arrival	Inpatient mortality rate
Coronary artery bypass graft	Aspirin at discharge Coronary artery bypass graft using internal mammary artery Prophylactic antibiotic within 1 hour of incision Appropriate prophylactic antibiotic selection Prophylactic antibiotic therapy ends within 24 hours of surgery end time	Inpatient mortality rate Postoperative bleeding or hematoma Postoperative physiologic or metabolic derangement
Heart failure	Left ventricular function assessment Detailed discharge instructions ACEI for left ventricular systolic dysfunction Smoking cessation advice/ counseling	
Community-acquired pneumonia	Percentage of patients who receive assessment of oxygenation within 24 hours of arrival Appropriate initial antibiotic Blood cultures before antibiotic administration Influenza screening/vaccination Antibiotic timing/% receiving antibiotics within 4 hours of arrival Smoking cessation advice/ counseling	
Hip and knee replacement	Prophylactic antibiotic received within 1 hour of incision Appropriate prophylactic antibiotic selection Prophylactic antibiotic stopped within 24 hours after surgery end time	Postoperative bleeding or hematoma Postoperative physiologic and metabolic derangement Readmissions 30 days after discharge

provide fewer services. These financial factors interplay with powerful nonfinancial motivations, such as professionalism, the desire to protect one's reputation among peers, and altruism. In this setting, it would be unwise to assume that new incentive programs, such as PR or PFP, will become the dominant determinants of behavior or will have any effect at all.[10]

Further complicating efforts to understand the impact of PR and PFP is the fact that the gold standard of research design, the randomized controlled trial, is rarely feasible for PR or PFP. It is unlikely that researchers would have the wherewithal to randomize communities to have a PR program in one arm and no PR program in the control arm. It is possible to observe whether consumers' choice of provider changes after reports about quality of care are released or whether providers' quality improvement efforts change after the introduction of PR. In terms of PFP, in some cases, providers can be randomized in PFP trials. In other cases, natural experiments have occurred; such as when a health plan that provides insurance in two different states introduces PFP in one state but not in the other. Before exploring the available evidence about PR and PFP, it may be useful to describe some key concepts in performance measurement.

Quality improvement efforts in other industries, and more recently in health care, have typically addressed three domains: structural, process, and outcome quality. In 1966, Donabedian[11] applied this framework to health care. In the health care context, structural quality refers to the resources available to deliver care—including equipment and human resources—and the physical environment in which care is delivered. Some examples of structural measures of care that have received significant attention recently are hospital and surgeon annual patient volume (on the assumption that higher volume translates to better quality) and availability of computerized physician order entry for inpatients (on the assumption that it will reduce medication errors). Process measures assess whether the appropriate care was delivered. An example would be to measure whether prophylactic antibiotics are given preoperatively and discontinued within a timely fashion. Finally, outcome quality is determined by changes in health status and is described as the end pathway of structural and process quality.[11] In this theoretic framework, poor process and structural quality should result in worse outcomes.

In general, outcome measures need to be risk adjusted, correcting an observed outcome rate to account for the severity of illness of each provider's or hospital's patient population. In general, process and structural measures do not require such adjustment. For almost all process measures, decision rules need to be developed to ensure that performance assessments only include patients for whom the measured process of care is truly appropriate.

PATIENT AND PROVIDER RESPONSES TO PUBLIC REPORTING

Previous PR efforts have targeted various combinations of the three domains of health care quality—structure, process, and outcome. This approach may have limited effects on quality improvement because patient and provider responses seem to vary depending on the specific aspect of quality measured and the level of public attention sought by the sponsors of the reports.[3,12] It is likely that a wide variation in what is being publicly reported coupled with differences in degree of public exposure and marketing of the information contribute to the fact that most of the studies described next have shown relatively small, albeit statistically significant, behavioral change in response to PR.

PR has been shown to influence patient choices. Multiple studies of consumer responses to health plan report cards show some impact of publicly reported health plan quality on health plan selection. There has been variation in the magnitude of the impact of public reports. In 1998, Chernew and Scanlon[13] showed that although report card ratings were related to enrollment choices, the relationship was neither linear nor uniform. Others have shown that other factors, not simply plan quality, have some influence on annual changes in enrollment.[14] One study of federal employees showed that health plan selection for newly hired employers was more influenced by quality scores than it was for long-term employees. The authors believed that this effect reflected long-term employees' access to other sources of information about the available health plans, including their own experiences and those of friends from the workplace. In this context, the report card actually added little new information to their decision-making process.[15] PR also has been shown to influence choice of physician in cardiac surgery. Mukamel and colleagues[16] found that PR was of greater importance to patients' surgeon choice than the surgeon's experience or the cost of care (although this was total cost, not just the portion borne by the patient). Overall, these documented effects have been limited; patients and referring providers are still often unaware of the breadth of information available or are just not using it to make provider selection or clinical decisions.[2,3]

Programs based on PR alone, targeted to practitioners, have been shown to increase quality improvement efforts within hospitals. In 2003, Hibbard and colleagues[17] showed that releasing hospital performance data publicly had a greater impact on hospitals' subsequent intensity of quality improvement efforts than providing the same information in a confidential report. This finding was especially true among hospitals whose performance was below average. In a subsequent study, Hibbard and colleagues[18] showed that even 2 years after release of a public report, a high percentage of consumers correctly identified hospitals that had done well, a potential for positive impact of PR systems. The theoretic incentives for improvement in this model are financial, because improved reputation may result in increased market share and institutional sustainability, and nonfinancial, with providers responding to concerns about their respective reputations or being driven by professional and altruistic motives and using the information to identify areas in which to improve.

It is also possible to do PR wrong, with the result that patients and providers largely ignore the data. For instance, for much of the 1980s, the Health Care Finance Agency (subsequently renamed CMS) released public reports of overall hospital mortality rates for all Medicare patients, with only minimal risk adjustment. Lack of clarity and transparency may have contributed to the lack of impact of the data on patient preferences, although it is possible that the patients simply believed that the data were not useful.[19] Providers also ignored the information, reporting that that they had little confidence in the validity of Health Care Finance Agency risk adjustment methodology.[20]

Although prior effects on individual consumers and providers have been relatively small, this could change over time. If PR and quality measurement become customary practice, we may reach a "tipping point" at which large proportions of consumers and providers are actively using the data as part of their usual approach to the health care system. With adequate transparency, consumer and provider confidence, and easy, ubiquitous accessibility, the impact of these programs might become significant. Based on this review of the literature, it is clear that the key to reaching this tipping point for PR involves acceptable risk adjustment and case mix metrics, user-friendly reports with succinct information, and successful marketing of the information.

IMPACT OF PAY-FOR-PERFORMANCE PROGRAMS

Although implementation of PFP programs in the United States has been relatively recent, some evidence suggests that if done right, it could improve clinical performance. Just as with PR, however, if designed incorrectly, programs could catalyze a significant attenuation of patient care and outcomes for some populations. In pediatrics, financial incentives—extra fees for each office visit that met a well-child or continuity of care goal—were convincingly linked to better care among resident physicians. Hickson and colleagues[21] showed that residents who were randomized to receive the incentive had better compliance with American Academy of Pediatrics' guidelines for well-child care, in part because they scheduled appointments above and beyond the Academy's recommendations.

Although PFP may improve process quality, the impact of these improvements on patient outcomes remains to be seen. A potential reason for a disconnection between processes and outcomes of care is that the first responses to the incentive may be administrative more than clinical. For example, pediatric immunizations were shown to improve in physicians randomized to receive fee-for-service or enhanced bonuses as compared with traditionally reimbursed practitioners.[22] On closer scrutiny, the rate of immunizations did not increase as much as documentation of immunization. Although it was not directly evaluated in the study, it is unlikely that patient outcomes improved as a result of better documentation in the absence of a true increase in the number of children immunized.

Mixed results were also reported in a study of tobacco cessation that compared multispecialty clinics randomized to receive financial incentives for reaching preset clinical performance targets and control clinics. Although increased referrals were observed in the financially incentivized clinics, the authors did not demonstrate a statistically significant difference in smoking cessation between the two groups.[23] Although these studies do not bolster the idea that successfully implemented PFP leads to better health outcomes, they do attest to the powerful influence of financial incentives on changing certain physician behaviors.

PUBLIC REPORTING AND PAY-FOR-PERFORMANCE: SUBSTITUTES OR COMPLEMENTS?

Few studies have compared the impact of PR to PFP. Available evidence suggests that they can work best when used together, however. In an early study of PR, Mehrotra and colleagues[12] interviewed hospital executives who had experienced local PR initiatives. Most executives reported that their institutions initially responded aggressively to having data about their performance released publicly. Many also reported that after several rounds of PR, if PFP or market share increases were not available, their hospital's commitment to responding to the public reports began to wane. In another study, Lindenauer and colleagues[24] assessed the effect of PFP plus PR versus PR alone on motivating quality improvement. The study showed a faster rate of overall improvement on overall quality measures at hospitals receiving PFP and PR than at facilities subject to PR alone. Taken together, these studies suggest that any emerging efforts to improve health care quality may be more successful if PR and PFP are used together.

UNINTENDED CONSEQUENCES OF PUBLIC REPORTING AND PAY-FOR-PERFORMANCE

Despite the documented potential for clinical benefit, it is also possible that PR and PFP, if implemented poorly, can cause harm. For instance, if physicians are not convinced that risk adjustment is adequate, they may attempt to game the system by avoiding patients they believe are at high risk for poor outcomes.[25] These unintended consequences may disproportionately impact specific subpopulations of patients and, depending on how rewards are allocated, programs may widen pre-existing quality gaps between physician groups. One piece of evidence for the potential detrimental effect of PR on access to care was noted in a survey of invasive cardiologists in Michigan and New York. In this study, most clinicians surveyed stated that PR affected their patient selection.[26] This finding suggests that concerns about risk-adjustment methods in PR programs could lead to decreased access to care and subsequent worsening of health outcomes for some already vulnerable populations.

Werner and colleagues[27,28] showed similar ill effects associated with New York State's cardiac surgery PR program. Werner and colleagues discovered that during the period after implementation of the program, African American patients experienced significant declines in access to cardiac surgical care. In Pennsylvania, however, cardiac surgical mortality rates and performance measurements were reported to surgeons confidentially but were not made public; there was no significant change in the baseline disparity. This finding suggests that patients who are perceived to be higher risk for surgery may be deselected under circumstances in which practitioners' reputation and potential market share depend on

distinctly measurable and quantifiable clinical outcomes, such as observed surgical mortality.

PUBLIC REPORTING AND PAY-FOR-PERFORMANCE IN THE SURGICAL SUBSPECIALTIES

Although there are a few PFP programs in the nascent phase at state and national levels, most of such programs focus on chronic disease and medical illnesses. This may reflect the relative dearth of surgeons within the organizations that develop performance measures for accreditation. Measures required for the accreditation of hospitals or health plans, many of which are already collected, have been the most readily available measures for PR and PFP. It also may be partly caused by the absence of appropriately trained surgeons participating in the development of quality measures. The quality of surgical care is difficult to measure. Few randomized controlled trials can unequivocally link process and structural measures to outcomes. A simple focus on surgical outcomes would be inappropriate, in many cases, because of uncertainties about how to adequately risk adjust those outcomes.

There is some limited experience with incentive-based programs in surgical subspecialties. These programs have been dominated by PR as opposed to PFP and have mainly been implemented in cardiac surgery.[29,30] Some PR in general surgery has focused on surgical site infections.[31] The remainder of this article focuses on PR and PFP in urologic surgery.

PUBLIC REPORTING AND PAY-FOR-PERFORMANCE IN UROLOGY: WHAT ARE THE OPTIONS?

Outside of efforts by insurers, there have been several attempts to develop quality indicators for assessing performance related to specific urologic procedures, such as radical prostatectomy. Investigators at the RAND Corporation have developed a set of detailed quality indicators for prostate cancer using a modified Delphi method.[32] Using a systematic and detailed literature review, patient focus groups, and expert interviews, RAND investigators led 11 members of an expert panel of urologists through a process in which they identified and then evaluated 44 candidate performance measures, including 5 structural indicators, 23 process measures, and 16 outcomes measures. The group concluded that there was not sufficient data to endorse any of the 5 structural measures. Patient satisfaction also was not endorsed as a quality indicator. The expert panel acknowledged that several of the indicators were not supported by published literature but nonetheless included some of these on the basis of logical relevance (eg, specialty board certification of providers, institutional tracking of outcomes and psychologic counseling). Of the 44 candidate indicators, the panel eventually endorsed 23 measures.

Miller and colleagues[33] subsequently conducted a retrospective review of hospital charts of 168 men who underwent prostate cancer therapy at the University of Michigan over a 5-year period to assess the feasibility of using the RAND quality of prostate cancer care measures and determine the associated changes in practice patterns. Of the 22 indicators included in the analysis, they reviewed the available data regarding compliance with 19 measures. They were unable to obtain data regarding compliance with 3 of the process indicators by chart review. Of the 19 process indicators for which compliance could be documented, 17 were evaluated by chart review, whereas 2 measures—pre- and posttreatment assessment of sexual, urinary, and bowel dysfunction—required access to their specific institutional database on prostate cancer patients. They were also able to document changes in compliance with several of the quality indicators over time. They concluded that it is feasible to measure compliance with the RAND urologic indicators using easily available, existing data sources and that these measures correlate with changes in prostate cancer treatment. The prostate cancer quality-of-care measures Miller and colleagues were able to evaluate are listed in **Box 1**.

Efforts at developing quality indicators for other urologic procedures are less mature as compared with prostate cancer; however, similar efforts are underway in bladder cancer. Several candidate measures have been proposed based on literature review.[34] No formal development or evaluation process has been undertaken by an academic or specialty urologic organization. **Box 2** lists potential candidate quality indicators for bladder cancer care, as suggested by Cooperberg and Konety.[34]

At the society level, the American Urologic Association, with the assistance of the American Medical Association, has constituted a panel to develop quality indicators for a wide variety of urologic diseases. This panel has developed a set of candidate measures for prostate cancer that are currently undergoing evaluation and ratification before being publicly released (David Penson, MD, personal communication, 2007). Three measures applicable to urology are included among the 74 measures in the 2007 Physician Quality Reporting Initiative supported by CMS. These measures include administration of antibiotics within 30 minutes to 1 hour of incision and venous

---

Box 1
RAND quality indicators for prostate cancer

Structural indicators

Number of patients treated (volume)

Availability of psychologic counseling

Knowledge of treating institution outcomes

Process indicators

Pretreatment prostate specific antigen (PSA), digital rectal examination, and Gleason sum

Documentation of pretreatment urinary, sexual, and bowel function

Assessment of family history of prostate cancer

Presentation of treatment alternatives, consultation with alternative providers, discussion of risks of therapy

Adherence to practice protocol of the College of American Pathologists Cancer Committee

At least two follow-up visits with treating physician in first year after therapy

Documentation of communication with primary care provider or provision of continuing care

Operative blood loss

Use of clinical and pathologic TNM staging

Outcome indicators

Primary treatment failure indicated by any detectable PSA after radical prostatectomy

After radical prostatectomy: hospitalization, medical or surgical treatment for bladder neck contracture/urethral stricture

Acute surgical complication rate

Patient assessment of urinary, sexual, and bowel function after radical prostatectomy using a validated survey instrument

Patient satisfaction with treatment choice, continence, and potency

Data from Miller DC, Litwin AS, Sanda MG, et al. Use of quality indicators to evaluate the care of patients with localized prostate carcinoma. Cancer 2003;97: 1428–35.

---

thromboembolism prophylaxis for a large majority of urologic operations. There is also a measure to assess the proportion of participating urologists who characterize and establish of a plan of care for urinary incontinence in female patients older than age 65.

In July 2007, CMS introduced the physician voluntary reporting program. In this program, physicians can voluntarily report selected quality

---

Box 2
Suggested performance measures for quality of bladder cancer care and radical cystectomy

Structure measures

Surgeon/hospital procedure volume

Availability of radiation therapy and chemotherapy services

Process measures

Time to cystectomy (< or > 3 months from diagnostic transuretheral resection of bladder tumor)

Adequacy of lymphadenectomy

Use (offer) of orthotopic urinary diversion

Appropriate use of neoadjuvant or adjuvant systemic chemotherapy

Outcome measures

Perioperative morbidity and mortality

Cancer-specific survival

Quality-of-life outcomes

Overall survival

Data from Cooperberg M, Konety BR. Quality of care indicators for radical cystectomy. In: Lee CT, Wood DP, editors. Bladder cancer: moving the field forward. Totowa (NJ): Humana Press Inc.; in press.

Box 3
Performance reporting codes used in the physician voluntary reporting programs sponsored by Centers for Medicare and Medicaid Services

CMS physician voluntary reporting program "G codes" for venous thromboembolism prophylaxis

G1855: Patient with documented receipt of thromboembolism prophylaxis

G1856: Patient without documented receipt of thromboembolism prophylaxis

G1857: Clinician documented that patient was not an eligible candidate for thromboembolism prophylaxis

Surgical site infection prevention

G1852: Patient documented to have received antibiotic prophylaxis 1 hour before incision time (2 hours for vancomycin)

G1853: Patient not documented to have received antibiotic prophylaxis 1 hour before incision time (2 hours for vancomycin)

G1854: Clinician documented that patient was not an eligible candidate for antibiotic prophylaxis 1 hour before incision time (2 hours for vancomycin)

Data from Centers for Medicare and Medicaid Services. Available at: http://www.cms.hhs.gov/Transmittals/downloads/R35DEMO.pdf. Page 19. Accessed September 10, 2008.

---

metrics using standard Medicare forms through "G codes" (**Box 3**). The two measures applicable to urology include venous thromboembolism prophylaxis and prevention of surgical site infection. Reporting on venous thromboembolism prophylaxis applies to a broad range of urologic procedures, which are too lengthy to list here, including procedures for benign and malignant conditions.[35] Reporting on surgical infection prevention applies to two specific urologic procedures: pelvic exenteration with/without hysterectomy, abdominoperineal resection and colostomy (CPT 51,597), and closure of rectovaginal fistula (CPT 57,307).

In contrast to the emphasis on quality measures in urologic malignancies by the American Urologic Association and CMS, some organizations, such as Hawaii Medical Services Association (the Hawaiian member of the national Blue Cross Blue Shield Association), have attempted to develop and implement process measures applicable to broader aspects of urologic practice including benign disease. Hawaii Medical Services Association's physician quality and service recognition program uses a point system to assess quality of urologic care in multiple dimensions. The dimensions used to compute a total score under the physician quality and service recognition include clinical quality indicators (40 points), patient satisfaction (20 points), business operations (20 points), and practice patterns (20 points). Awards for meeting performance standards varied between 3% and 7.5% of baseline physician fee-for-service payments from the prior year. This translated into $500 to $16,000 per provider in 2004.[36] **Table 3** lists the quality measures used to assess urologic care in this program. Many of these measures are based on acknowledged standards of clinical practice. Not all are equally supported by clinical evidence as having a positive impact on outcomes, however. Because the program is relatively new, the impact of this PFP initiative is not yet known. The Hawaii Medical Services Association is also working with physicians to evaluate potential approaches to actually improving quality. The impact on changes in practice patterns remains to be seen because there has been little evaluative research to date.

There are always pitfalls in developing comprehensive measures to gauge clinical performance,

Table 3
Hawaii Medical Services Association quality indicators for urological care[36]

Quality Indicator	Metric
Follow-up after diagnosis of prostate cancer	Obtaining at least one PSA level in first year after diagnosis of prostate cancer
Initial evaluation of hematuria	Upper tract study, cytology, cystoscopy for patients with risk factors or age > 40
Liver function tests (LFTs) for patients on bicalutamide (Casodex)	Patients who had at least one set of LFTs obtained within 90 days of first (index) of two separately dated prescriptions for bicalutamide (Casodex)
Urine culture before antibiotic administration for female patients with urinary tract infection visiting urologists	Women filling a prescription for an antibiotic written by a urologist who received a urinalysis or urine culture within 7 days before filling the prescription
Use of semen analysis, prostatic smear, or prostate biopsy in diagnostic evaluation of patients with chronic prostatitis	Patients undergoing a prostatic smear, semen analysis, urinalysis, urine culture, or prostate biopsy 1 month before and 2 months after diagnosis of chronic prostatitis
Use of short-course antibiotic therapy in women with uncomplicated urinary tract infection	Women with a diagnosis of urinary tract infection given a 3-day antibiotic prescription; antibiotic type is specified as part of measure

especially if the data supporting such measures are not based on class I evidence. For example, one of the quality measures used in the Hawaii Medical Services Association performance assessment is conducting a PSA test each year in patients with a primary diagnosis of prostate cancer. It is unclear from the measure description if only newly diagnosed cases are included in the annual assessment. Currently, most urologists use PSA testing routinely in the follow-up of patients with prostate cancer. The ideal or most cost-efficient protocol for PSA follow-up testing in patients who have prostate cancer has not been determined. In general, the test is performed more frequently during the first few years after diagnosis, and the frequency is reduced to yearly in patients who are more than 5 years after diagnosis. Hypothetically, a patient who is 5 years posttreatment and who has shown no signs of recurrence may undergo PSA testing at intervals longer than 1 year with no untoward clinical consequences. The associated provider might be judged to be noncompliant with this measure, however, and may receive diminished reimbursement. The literature most often cited as evidence for the use of this measure pertains to a specific subpopulation of patients with hormone refractory prostate cancer.

SUMMARY

Currently, whether PR and PFP programs improve the quality of care has yet to be determined;

however, PR and PFP programs are being rapidly implemented across the country. It is likely that many urologists will find their performance being measured in PR and PFP programs soon if it is not already being done. As the RAND study demonstrated, however, there is a lack of class I data to support many proposed quality indicators in urology. Some indicators still may be important based on logical relevance to urologic practice. This fact underscores the importance of specialist participation in determining indicators for PR because logical relevance can best be determined by experienced appropriately trained providers. This specialty-specific expertise and participation also will be useful to predict how potential pitfalls and adverse reactions to incentive-based programs, such as system gaming and deselection of high-risk patients, can be avoided.

Input from urologists in the development of PFP programs is crucial in determining the most effective ways to administer financial incentives. For example, appropriately trained and experienced urologists are in the best position to comment on the debate about whether bonuses should be distributed based on reaching set standard benchmarks or on demonstration of improvement over time. Although PR and PFP programs are rapidly evolving, nationwide implementation of broadspectrum urology practice measures of quality has yet to occur. Efforts by the American Urologic Association in collaboration with the American Medical Association represent a solid start to defining what should be measured and rewarded as a reflection of quality in urologic care. To maximize efficiency and quality while avoiding detrimental affects to the patients, it behooves urologists and other specialists to provide leadership in the initial design and subsequent evolution of these programs.

REFERENCES

1. United States Health and Human Services. Available at: www.hhs.gov/transparency/index.html. Accessed May 30, 2007.
2. Schneider EC, Epstein AM. Influence of cardiac-surgery performance reports on referral practices and access to care: a survey of cardiovascular specialists. N Engl J Med 1996;335(4):251–6.
3. Schneider EC, Epstein AM. Use of public performance reports: a survey of patients undergoing cardiac surgery. JAMA 1998;279(20):1638–42.
4. Schneider EC, Lieberman T. Publicly disclosed information about the quality of health care: response of the US public. Qual Health Care 2001;10(2):96–103.
5. Integrated Healthcare Association. Advancing quality through collaboration: a compendium of California healthcare quality improvement projects. Available at: http://www.iha.org/rchrpt/lha%20v7%20final.pdf. Accessed May 28, 2007.
6. The Leapfrog Group for Patient Safety. Available at: http://ir.leapfroggroup.org/compendium/. Accessed July 18, 2007.
7. Blue Cross Premier Program. Available at: http://www.premierinc.com/about/mission. Accessed July 16, 2007.
8. Centers for Medicare and Medicaid Services. Rewarding superior quality care: the premier hospital quality incentive demonstration. March 2005. Available at: http://www.premierinc.com/quality-safety/tools-services/p4p/hqi/resources/clinical-conditions-and-measures-effective-7-1-2005-discharges.pdf. Accessed October 10, 2008.
9. Frolich A, Talavera JA, Broadhead P, et al. A behavioral model of clinician responses to incentives to improve quality [review]. Health Policy 2007;80(1):179–93 [Epub 2006 Apr 19].
10. Rosenthal MB, Frank RG. What is the empirical basis for paying for quality in health care? Med Care Res Rev 2006;63(2):135–7.
11. Donabedian A. Evaluating the quality of medical care 1966. Milbank Q 2005;83(4):691–729.
12. Mehrotra A, Lee S, Dudley RA. Hospital performance evaluation: what data do we want, how do we get it, and how should we use it? Presented at the National Business Coalition on Health Conference. Chicago, June 16–17, 2003.
13. Chernew M, Scanlon DP. Health plan report cards and insurance choice. Inquiry 1998;35(1):9–22.
14. Beaulieu ND. Quality information and consumer health plan choices. J Health Econ 2002;21(1):43–63.
15. Wedig GJ, Tai Seale M. The effect of report cards on consumer choice in the health insurance market. J Health Econ 2002;21(6):1031–48.
16. Mukamel DB, Weimer DL, Zwanziger J, et al. Quality report cards, selection of cardiac surgeons, and racial disparities: a study of the publication of the New York state cardiac surgery reports. Inquiry 2004,2005;41(4):435–46.
17. Hibbard JH, Stockard J, Tusler M. Does publicizing hospital performance stimulate quality improvement efforts? Health Aff (Millwood) 2003;22(2):84–94.
18. Hibbard JH, Stockard J, Tusler M. It isn't just about choice: the potential of a public performance report to affect the public image of hospitals. Med Care Res Rev 2005;62(3):358–71.
19. Vladeck BC, Goodwin EJ, Myers LP, et al. Consumers and hospital use: the HCFA "death list." Health Aff (Millwood) 1988;7(1):122–5.
20. Berwick DM, Wald DL. Hospital leaders' opinions of the HCFA mortality data. JAMA 1990;263(2):247–9.
21. Hickson GB, Altemeier WA, Perrin JM. Physician reimbursement by salary or fee-for-service: effect on physician practice behavior in a randomized prospective study. Pediatrics 1987;80(3):344–50.
22. Fairbrother G, Hanson KL, Friedman S, et al. The impact of physician bonuses, enhanced fees and feedback on childhood immunization coverage rates. Am J Public Health 1999;89(2):171–5.
23. Roski J, Jeddeloh R, An L, et al. The impact of financial incentives and a patient registry on preventive care quality: increasing provider adherence to evidence-based smoking cessation practice guidelines. Prev med 2003;36(3):291–9.
24. Lindenauer PK, Remus D, Roman S, et al. Public reporting and pay-for-performance in hospital quality improvement. N Engl J Med 2007;356(5):486–96.
25. Petersen LA, Woodard LD, Urech T, et al. Does pay-for-performance improve the quality of healthcare? Ann Intern Med 2006;145(4):265–72.
26. No authors. Study raises concerns on public reporting of data. Healthcare Benchmarks Qual Improv 2005;12(8):88–9.
27. Werner RM, Asch DA, Polsky D. Racial profiling: the unintended consequences of coronary artery bypass graft report cards. Circulation 2006;111(10):1257–63.
28. Werner RM, Asch DA. The unintended consequences of publicly reporting quality information. JAMA 2005;293(10):1239–44.
29. Hannan EL, Kumar D, Racz M, et al. New York State's cardiac surgery reporting system: four years later. Ann Thorac Surg 1994;58(6):1852–7.
30. Shahian DM, Normad SL, Torchiana DF, et al. Cardiac surgery report cards: comprehensive review and statistical critique. Ann Thorac Surg 2001;72(6):2155–68.

31. Bratzler DW. The surgical infection prevention and surgical care improvement projects: promises and pitfalls. Am Surg 2006;72(11):1010–6 [discussion: 1021–30, 1133–48].

32. Spencer BA, Steinberg M, Malin J. Quality-of-care indicators for early-stage prostate cancer. J Clin Oncol 2003;21(10):1928–36.

33. Miller DC, Litwin AS, Sanda MG, et al. Use of quality indicators to evaluate the care of patients with localized prostate carcinoma. Cancer 2003;97:1428–35.

34. Cooperberg M, Konety BR. Quality of care indicators for radical cystectomy. In: Lee CT, Wood DP, editors. Bladder cancer: moving the field forward. Totowa (NJ): Humana Press Inc.; in press.

35. Centers for Medicare and Medicaid Services. Available at: http://www.cms.hhs.gov/apps/media/. Accessed August 9, 2007.

36. Chung RS, Chernicoff HO, Nakao KA. A quality driven physician compensation model: four-year follow-up study. J Healthc Qual 2003;25(6):31–7.

American Health Care at the Crossroads

Newt Gingrich, David Merritt*

KEYWORDS

- Individual health • Culture of health • Delivery of care
- Financing of health insurance

American health care has reached a fork in the road. The current path, littered with waste, rising costs, and errors, leaves Americans no choice but to change. There is a positive way forward. Health and health care can be transformed. Americans can become healthier individuals and control costs. Quality can be improved. One hundred percent insurance coverage can be obtained. But to succeed it will take bold, transformational, and collaborative solutions.

That is what the Center for Health Transformation[1] is devoted to creating: a 21st century intelligent health system that brings more choices of greater quality at lower costs to every American. And there are things that must be done as a country, as communities, as companies, and as individuals to get there.

WHY BOLDNESS IS NEEDED

The nation spends a staggering amount of money on health care. Just to put the size and scope of the health care system in context, think of it this way. Last year the United States spent $2 trillion—16 percent of the economy—on health care. This is almost the entire gross domestic product of France, Britain, or China; it almost doubles the entire economy of Canada. Just

what Americans spend on health care is larger than the gross domestic product of 175 nations.[†]

And health care costs continue to rise. According to the Centers for Medicare and Medicaid Services (CMS), last year was a good year, when health care costs rose only 6.8 percent.[2] CMS projects that within the decade, by 2016, total health care spending will more than double to $4.1 trillion a year and consume 19.6 percent of United States gross domestic product.[3] The country cannot sustain its current path.

States are not immune from the burden of health care. Both as employers and as insurers through the State Children's Health Insurance Program (SCHIP) and Medicaid, states pay the price of the current system. For example, Florida spends about 25 percent of its budget on Medicaid. Former Florida Governor Jeb Bush told at the Center for Health Transformation that if nothing changes, 10 years from now Medicaid will consume 59 percent of all state revenue. This will crowd out every other priority, including education, transportation, law enforcement, and others. States cannot sustain this current path.

Individuals fare no better, despite the incredible amount of money spent on health care every year. Key quality indicators continue to show little improvement, and some even show decline. The rates of obesity and diabetes are increasing

[†]The Center for Health Transformation, founded and led by former Speaker of the House Newt Gingrich, is a collaboration of leaders dedicated to the creation of a 21st century intelligent health system that saves lives and saves money for all United States citizens. Center members highlighted in this testimony include Microsoft, Intermountain Healthcare, WellPoint, IBM, UnitedHealth Group, UPS, WellStar Health System, Georgia Hospital Association, AT&T, Southern Company, American Academy of Family Physicians, and Blue Cross Blue Shield of Georgia. For more information on The Center for Health Transformation, please visit www.healthtransformation.net.
Former Speaker of the House Newt Gingrich is the founder of the Center for Health Transformation. David Merritt is a project director at the Center.
Center for Health Transformation, The Gingrich Group, 1425 K Street, Northwest, Suite 450, Washington, DC 20005, USA
* Corresponding author.
E-mail address: dmerritt@gingrichgroup.com (D. Merritt).

Urol Clin N Am 36 (2009) 49–55
doi:10.1016/j.ucl.2008.08.010

rapidly, and the real threat of preventable medical errors remains a dangerous reality for millions of Americans. According to the Institute of Medicine, individuals average one medication error every day they stay in a hospital—1.5 million medication errors every year.[4] More than 7,000 Americans are killed every year from preventable medication errors, and up to 98,000 Americans are killed every year by preventable medical errors.[5] And that is likely a very conservative estimate.

According to the Kaiser Family Foundation, between 2000 and 2007, health insurance premiums skyrocketed 87 percent. Over the same period, inflation rose by 18 percent, and wages grew by only 20 percent.[6] In addition, the number of Americans without health insurance is also on the rise. According to a recent report by the Census Bureau, a record 47 million Americans lack health insurance.[7]

Many policymakers, journalists, and industry leaders try to group all 47 million people into the same category. This assumes, incorrectly, that everyone without insurance is in this predicament for the same reason, when in fact there are three distinct groups with far different reasons for being uninsured.

The first group consists of Americans who are uninsured but earn more than $50,000 a year. According to the same Census Bureau report, there are 15 million Americans who lack insurance but earn more than $50,000 a year—eight million of whom earn more than $75,000 a year. According to a 2003 study by the Congressional Budget Office (CBO), nearly 11 percent of the uninsured were so because they did not believe in insurance or "have not needed insurance."[8] Many in this group choose not to purchase health insurance.

The second group is made up of individuals who do not have health insurance, because they have moved, lost a job, or their employer does not offer coverage anymore. Many in this group ultimately get coverage. The CBO estimated that 45 percent of those without insurance lack coverage for less than 4 months.[8]

The third group consists of people who are chronically uninsured and are, in essence, locked out of the system. They were denied coverage or simply cannot afford or were not offered health insurance through their employer, but they earn too much to qualify for a public program.

Regardless of how or why someone is uninsured, to walk in his or here shoes can be a sad situation. These individuals have virtually no access to a primary care doctor, will likely be sicker, and may die needlessly. The Institute of Medicine estimates that the lack of health insurance leads to the deaths of 18,000 Americans every year.[9] They often live in fear every day. Fear that their child will get sick but cannot see a doctor. Fear that their spouse will have a serious accident that prevents him or her from working. And the constant fear that they are one step away from medical bankruptcy.[10]

The plight of the uninsured affects every citizen—even those who are insured. Every individual who has health insurance pays a hidden tax to cover the cost of delivering care to the uninsured. After all, people without insurance still need and ultimately do get medical care, but it is often in an emergency department, the most expensive health care setting one can find. The cost of this care is passed along to those who have insurance in the form of higher insurance premiums. Ken Thorpe of Emory University estimates that in 2010 these higher premiums for those with insurance will total more than $60 billion—more than $1,500 in hidden costs for every insured family.[11] Individuals and families simply cannot sustain this current path.

Such failure cannot be accepted. Coverage can be extended to all Americans, but it will take bold, transformational solutions. This requires collaboration, consensus, and action from everyone—from employers, providers, insurers, and citizens, to policymakers of both parties.

What presidential candidates, trade associations, think tanks, governors, and others have proposed so far, however, is typically more of the same tired financing that has been seen many times before. Most plans focus exclusively on coverage, and while that is an essential focus of any solution, they try to cover the uninsured within the current system. This is akin to building a house on quicksand. These plans have nary a word on how to make health care more affordable, and that is why they will all fail.

The uninsured crisis is a symptom of the larger structural problem of rising health care costs. As in medicine, one must cure the disease, not just alleviate its symptoms. By driving down costs and making health care more affordable for every American, 100 percent coverage can be achieved. But to get there, four transformational changes must be implemented:

> Improve individual health
> Create a culture of health
> Modernize and improve the delivery of care
> Transform the financing of health insurance

IMPROVE INDIVIDUAL HEALTH

First, one must focus on health—then health care—and individuals must take an active role in becoming healthier. The Centers for Disease Control and Prevention (CDC) report that

64 percent of adults are either overweight or obese.[12] The CDC also reported that diabetes is a major factor in killing more than 220,000 Americans every year.[13] These two conditions alone cost the system hundreds of billions of dollars every year. But they are, for the most part, a consequence of poor individual choices. Individuals must be incentivized to improve their health and prevent disease by making more responsible decisions. This can be done through closer relationships with their physicians, proper education, and through wellness programs that reward healthy living.

For example, Blue Cross Blue Shield of Michigan introduced Healthy Blue Living, where individuals can save 10 percent or more on their premiums, copayments, and deductibles if they work with their physician, exercise, eat right, control chronic conditions, and do not smoke.

Under former Governor Jeb Bush, Florida Medicaid introduced a new approach to incentivize beneficiaries to focus on their health. Medicaid members could earn credits, up to $125 in value, if they met certain goals, such as preventive care maintenance, immunizations, and completing health screenings.

United Healthcare has introduced a product called Vital Measures, where individuals with a high-deductible health plan coupled with a Health Savings Account can earn up to $2,000 toward their annual deductible of $2,500 if they meet certain health benchmarks.

These examples are the exception, not the rule. State and federal laws often stand in the way of making these types of plans the norm. State and federal rules, Heath Insurance Portability and Accountability Act (HIPAA) most notably, must be reformed to give private health plans, including those that participate in Medicaid and Medicare, more latitude to design insurance products to encourage and reward individual healthy behaviors.

New models of care and payment that make health and wellness a priority must be established. The American Academy of Family Physicians and others have advocated the medical home model. This approach strengthens the doctor–patient relationship by focusing both the consumer and the physician on improving individual health. Primary care physicians deliver care that focuses on wellness, early intervention, and the prevention of chronic illness, in addition to acute illness, as necessary. In addition to this focus on wellness, another hallmark of the medical home concept is for physicians to help coordinate the services that consumers receive in other sectors of the health system.

North Carolina's Medicaid program spent $20 million in payments to 3,500 primary care physicians who transformed their practices to participate in a medical home pilot. Through reduced hospitalizations, better control of chronic disease, and the reduction of complications, this investment saved Medicaid more than $231 million in 2005 and 2006.

Consumers also must have the tools with which to better manage their health. The use of personal health records can be portals to health education, cost and quality data, and personal health histories. These kinds of online tools can bring to health care the kind of consumer technology available in every other aspect of life. Personal health records can deliver:

Wellness and education content
Better understanding of treatment options
Connectivity with doctors
Unlimited online access to personal health information
Cost and performance data on physicians, hospitals, and insurers
Emergency information, such as family contacts, allergies, current medications, and medical history

The Wall Street Journal released a survey that asked, "Which of the following technologies would you like to have access to when seeking care from a doctor or hospital?" Seventy-four percent of respondents said they would like to use E-mail to communicate directly with their doctor; 75 percent said they would like the ability to schedule a doctor's visit online. Sixty-seven percent said they would like to receive the results of diagnostic tests by E-mail, and 77 percent said they would like to receive E-mail reminders from their doctors.[14]

But when asked if they had access to these services, most consumers said they did not. Ninety-two percent of the public cannot E-mail their doctor; 93 percent cannot schedule an appointment online. Ninety-five percent of consumers cannot get their laboratory results online, 93 percent do not receive E-mail reminders from their doctors.

When it comes to information technology, consumers are ready, but the system is not. From Microsoft to health insurers to physician-driven portals, public and private institutions must find effective ways to engage consumers to improve their health. And technology can play an important role.

It is only through engaging individuals to become healthier will health begin to be transformed. The kind of change needed cannot be brought about if health indicators continue to stagnate and decline. It is a recipe for higher costs and poorer health.

CREATE A CULTURE OF HEALTH

A culture of health must be created that encourages more responsible individual choices. This can be done by redesigning how public and private institutions influence individual behavior, and nowhere is this needed more than in public education.

The CDC reports that nearly 80 percent of students—40 million of them—do not eat the recommended five servings of fruits and vegetables a day, and only one in three high school students participates in daily physical education.[15] Nearly half of America's youth, aged 12 to 21 years, are not vigorously active on a regular basis.[16] It should come as no surprise then that the number of obese children has tripled since 1980.[17] This, however, can be corrected with smart policies that give children an encouraging environment to be more active and choose healthier foods.

For instance, physical education five days a week should be required for every student in grades kindergarten through 12. Individual student health reports, including weight and body mass index, should be collected and sent home to parents, along with relevant educational material. School lunches, breakfasts, and vending machines should promote healthy foods, so that unhealthy alternatives are penalized or prohibited. The University of Virginia Health System has an innovative program that prices and color codes snacks according to their health value in all vending machines and cafeterias.[18]

Another example is Somerville, Massachusetts. This community should be a model for all others to follow to promote individual health, particularly that of children. In 2002, 46 percent of Somerville's first through third graders were either at-risk of becoming overweight or already were overweight.[19] With the specter of serious health implications looming down the road, the community came together, from teachers, school officials, and parents, to restaurant owners, city government, nurses, and physicians. They created the "Shape Up Somerville" program, which was a three-year initiative that sought to prevent obesity in first, second, and third grade students.

Specific changes included:

Improving school cafeteria menus
Food education at both school and at home
Before-, during-, and after-school curriculum that was modified to promote health, activity, and nutrition
Restaurants modified their menus to be "shape up approved"
New bike and walking paths were constructed within a half-mile of schools
Education and training toolkits for community nurses and physicians were created to educate providers on the best approaches to treat childhood obesity

In just one year, the rate of overweight students started coming down.

Outside of public education, there are other community-based changes that could create a culture of health. Grocery stores should receive tax incentives to open in urban areas if they provide a wide selection of fresh fruits and vegetables. (The city of Detroit does not have a single national grocery chain operating within city limits.) The federal government should redesign the food stamp and Women Infants and Children (WIC) programs to incentivize the purchase of healthier foods. State and local governments should invest in bike paths, sidewalks, public parks, and active recreation programs to encourage physical activity. And consumers need tools to be better educated on their choices, as Safeway has done by creating an online portal called FoodFlex. This site allows consumers to view a personalized history of the foods that they purchased, with tips and recommendations on nutrition and healthier alternatives.

Employers can use the workplace to create a culture of health and influence better individual decisions. Not only do healthier employees enjoy a better quality of life, but they are very good business. IBM has more than 40 wellness programs that address health promotion, industrial hygiene and safety, medical management, and benefit design. These programs have reduced emergency room visits by as much as 24 percent and hospital admissions by as much as 37 percent.[20] Researchers in the *American Journal of Health Promotion* reviewed 73 studies of similar worksite health promotion programs and concluded that employers had an average return of nearly $4 to $1.[21]

These kinds of changes can play an important role in creating an environment that encourages individuals to make better decisions about their health.

IMPROVE AND MODERNIZE THE DELIVERY OF CARE

How people receive care once they are in the health care system must be improved and modernized dramatically. This must start with rooting out waste and inefficiencies. Dr. Brent James of Intermountain Healthcare and Dr. Robert Brook of RAND Health, both members of the Institute of Medicine, estimate that at least one-third—and perhaps as much as half—of all spending in health care is waste, or adds no value to the clinic process.

One of the most important changes is to eliminate any financial incentive to do any test, treatment, or therapy that does not directly benefit the patient or add value to the care process. The surest way to accomplish this is to change the physician or hospital payments from a transaction-based to an outcomes-based model.

The current payment system simply is based on the number of transactions or services that are provided, regardless of their necessity, value, or quality of care. This approach has an inherent incentive for the overuse of resources. Those and physicians who deliver better care for the most part are reimbursed at the exact same rate as those who provide poorer care.

A new model is needed. Reimbursement will drive change, be it using a new test, device, or treatment, and a model is needed that takes into account the quality of the care that is delivered.

Changing what is paid for will encourage the use of new tools, techniques, and technologies that will lead to better care. This kind of change is vital, as providers have yet to adopt new technology or adhere to clinical guidelines en masse on their own.

For example, the adoption of health information technology, such as electronic health records, computerized physician order entry, and electronic prescribing, remains abysmal, despite the fact that these technologies have been available for years, and much evidence and research proves their effectiveness and efficiency. Take electronic prescribing. This technology can replace handwritten, misread, and mismatched prescriptions with online, automated, and expert technology. Physicians know this technology saves lives and money. According to a recent survey of 400 physicians, 81 percent of physicians say the widespread use of electronic prescribing would reduce medication errors; 85 percent of physicians think electronic prescribing is a good idea, and 65 percent say it would save time.

Despite knowing its benefits, only 7 percent of physicians actually use the technology, and almost two out of three say implementing electronic prescribing is not a priority for their practice. The number one reason? It is not in their financial interest.[22]

Fundamentally changing the way providers are paid can correct this. Current pay-for-performance and other incentive programs are a first step toward an outcomes-based payment structure.

CMS and many private insurers are partnering with their physician and hospital networks to pilot new financing and delivery models based on outcomes, from the Leapfrog Group and Integrated Healthcare Association to Blue Cross Blue Shield plans and Bridges to Excellence. All of them know that reimbursement drives adoption.

In Georgia, the Center for Health Transformation is leading the nation's largest Bridges to Excellence diabetes program. Led by UPS, AT&T, and Southern Company— all members of the Center for Health Transformation—there are currently 14 major employers, including the state of Georgia, participating in the program. The state medical society and hospital association are participating actively also. Serving in the role of administrators are Blue Cross Blue Shield of Georgia, Humana, Aetna, CIGNA, Kaiser Permanente, and UnitedHealthcare. Physician recruitment efforts are ongoing, with WellStar Health System and the Morehouse Community Physician Network leading the way.

The program, like other pay-for-performance initiatives, pays incentives to physicians who practice best standards of diabetes care. The program encourages individuals who have diabetes to see these physicians to improve their quality of life and avoid the long-term complications of the disease. In the process, physicians are rewarded for providing high-quality care; individuals with diabetes are healthier, and employers save money. A recent actuarial analysis of the program by Towers Perrin reports an estimated savings of $1,059 per individual if blood pressure, hemoglobin A1C, and low-density lipoprotein (LDL) control measures are met. By saving lives and saving money, this Bridges to Excellence module should be the minimum standard of diabetic care throughout the country.

Other examples of new reimbursement approaches include health insurers Aetna and CIGNA Healthcare. In select markets, they will reimburse physicians for conducting electronic or Web-based consultations with their patients. Physicians in Ohio and New Hampshire are working with WellPoint, the nation's largest insurer, to implement electronic prescribing. WellPoint is covering part of the hardware and service costs, and reimbursing doctors using E-prescribing at a higher rate than those still writing paper prescriptions.

Federal officials are moving in this direction also. The Center for Health Transformation has partnered with Senator John Kerry on using payment incentives to drive use of electronic prescribing— along with a federal requirement in Medicare if adoption is slow.[23] In November 2007, the American Health Information Community, an advisory body to Health and Human Services (HHS) Secretary Mike Leavitt, agreed to recommend this model in federal programs.

CMS began an innovative initiative called the Medicare Health Care Quality Demonstration Program, also known as the 646 demonstrations. A major focus of these five-year demonstrations is to improve the delivery of care in ambulatory offices by testing significant changes to payment and reimbursement, and performance measures and the practice of evidence-based medicine. These demonstrations should provide valuable insights for specifics models to introduce more broadly.

Tying reimbursement to improve outcomes will encourage physician adoption of the tools, techniques, and technologies that will deliver better care.

TRANSFORM THE FINANCING OF HEALTH INSURANCE

The way health insurance is financed also must be changed radically. Between individuals and their doctors are mountains of burdensome regulations, hoards of middlemen, and red tape as far as the eye can see. In no other sector of society does one accept such a convoluted approach to buying a product or service. Putting consumers squarely in control is essential.

One of the most important changes that can be made is to give consumers the right to purchase a health insurance policy from anywhere in the country.

Current state and federal laws permit consumers to buy only those health insurance plans that have been approved in their own state, meaning it is illegal for a citizen of one state to buy insurance in another. These government barriers to free trade stifle competition, producing disastrous results. The absence of robust competition artificially inflates the cost of insurance, preventing millions of citizens from purchasing affordable coverage.

To reverse this, government must allow competition to flourish. More competition among insurers in a nationwide market will encourage more creative products, better services and lower prices—just as it always does wherever competition thrives—and every American will be able to find affordable coverage. More competition and consumer empowerment will go a long way toward creating a free, fair, and functional marketplace in health care.

A vital part of a functional market is the availability of information. Information on performance, cost, and quality allows consumers to make informed decisions, but health care is perhaps the only market in which consumers have virtually no access to this information. When Americans shop for a new car, home, or thousands of other items, they quickly and easily gather information on cost and quality from an endless array of resources. But in health care, consumers are virtually blind. Try finding out how a doctor stacks up

against his colleagues. Try finding out how much a hospital charges for an elective surgery. Try finding out which surgical team has the lowest mortality rate.

Americans have a right to know this information, Medicare claims history can provide that data best. Medicare has detailed information on nearly every doctor and hospital in the country, which can be analyzed to identify the most efficient hospitals, best doctors, and most effective treatments. The federal government also has information on disciplinary action and lawsuits filed against physicians, collected for the National Practitioner Data Bank. Inexplicably and inexcusably, the federal government will not release this data.

Despite growing demands from many health plans, employers, consumers, and researchers—even an ongoing lawsuit where HHS has appealed a federal judge's ruling to release the Medicare data—this information remains locked away from taxpayers. This information will save lives and save money now. Americans have a right to know this information, and taxpayers must continue to demand its release.[24]

The individual should be empowered to root out waste by creating incentives for consumers to pursue better care at lower cost, so the citizen becomes the primary driver of cost reduction in health care. Consumers should have the right to purchase insurance policies that are tailored to their specific needs. And individuals who purchase their own insurance should receive the same tax benefits as employers who provide coverage.

Finally, information-rich health savings accounts should be available to everyone, regardless of how or whether they obtain insurance, and consumers should be able to pay health insurance premiums with health savings account dollars.

SUMMARY

All of these solutions are fundamental changes from today's approach to health care. But to build a 21st century intelligent health system, embracing this level of change is an absolute necessity.

These kinds of changes will break a lot of china. They represent a serious effort that can improve quality, reduce health care costs, and expand insurance coverage—things that the current system is incapable of doing. Today's system will result in rising costs, poor quality, too many without insurance, and an unhealthy population. Any plan to cover the uninsured that builds upon such a dysfunctional system simply throws good money after bad.

We can do better.

With real change, through the ideas outlined in this article, individual health can be improved, modernize the delivery and administration of care modernized, and insurance to every American expanded. Americans deserve nothing less.

REFERENCES

1. World Bank. World development indicators database. July 2007.
2. Poisal JA, Truffer C, Smith S, et al. Health spending projections through 2016: modest changes obscure part D's impact. Health Aff 2007;26:w242–53.
3. Centers for Medicare and Medicaid Services. Office of the Actuary. National health expenditure projections 2006–2016. 2006.
4. Institute of Medicine. Preventing medication errors. 2006.
5. Institute of Medicine. To err is human. 2000.
6. Kaiser Family Foundation and the Health Research and Educational Trust, Employer Health Benefits: 2006 survey.
7. US Census Bureau. Income, poverty, and health insurance coverage in the United States: 2006. August 2007.
8. Congressional Budget Office. How many people lack health insurance and for how long? May 2003.
9. Institute of Medicine. Insuring America's health: principles and recommendations. January, 2004.
10. Gingrich N, Merritt D. One cheer for Doctor Hillary. National Review Online. October 15, 2007.
11. Thorpe K. Paying a premium: the added cost of care for the uninsured. Families USA Publication 2005; 5–101.
12. Centers for Disease Control and Prevention. National Health and Nutrition Examination Survey, healthy weight, overweight, and obesity among US adults. July 2003. Available at: http://www.cdc.gov/nchs/data/nhanes/databriefs/adultweight.pdf.
13. Centers for Disease Control and Prevention. National diabetes fact sheet. Available at: http://www.cdc.gov/diabetes/pubs/factsheet.htm. 2003.
14. Harris Interactive Poll. Wall Street Journal Online September 2006.
15. Centers for Disease Control and Prevention. Healthy youth: an investment in our nation's future. 2007.
16. Office of the Surgeon General of the United States. Physical activity and health: adolescents and young adults. 1999.
17. Centers for Disease Control and Prevention. National Center for Health Statistics. Prevalence of overweight among children and adolescents: United States, 1999–2002. 2004.
18. Garson Arthur Jr, Engelhard Carolyn L. Attacking obesity: lessons from smoking. J Am Coll Cardiol 2007;49:1673–5.
19. Available at: http://nutrition.tufts.edu/.
20. Barlow JF. Testimony before the House Government Reform Committee, Subcommittee on Federal Workforce and Agency Organization, March 15, 2006.
21. Aldana SG. Financial impact of health promotion programs: a comprehensive review of the literature. Am J Health Promot 2001;15(5):296–320.
22. Ayres, McHenry, et al. On behalf of the Pharmaceutical Care Management Association. Survey of physicians regarding E-prescribing, July 2007.
23. Kerry J, Gingrich N. E-prescriptions. Wall St J 2007.
24. Gingrich N, Merritt D. Renew Milton Friedman's conservatism. National Review Online. December 4, 2006.

US Health Care: Single-Payer or Market Reform

David U. Himmelstein, MD, Steffie Woolhandler, MD, MPH*

KEYWORDS

- Health insurance • Access to care • Health policy
- Single-payer health care

Almost all agree that our health care system is dysfunctional. Forty-seven million Americans have no health insurance, resulting in more than 18,000 unnecessary deaths annually according to the Institute of Medicine.[1] Tens of millions more have inadequate coverage. Health care costs reached $7498 per capita this year, 50% higher than in any other nation, and continue to grow rapidly. Market pressures threaten medicine's best traditions, and bureaucracy overwhelms doctors and patients. Opinion on solutions is more divided.

Discussion of health reform was muted in the 1990s after the defeat of President Clinton's Byzantine scheme for universal coverage. Now, however, the accelerating collapse of employment-based coverage under the pressure of globalization is reopening debate. Firms like General Motors and Ford are crippled by the growing burden of health costs, which add $1500 to the price of a General Motors car versus $419 for a German Mercedes and $97 for a Japanese Toyota.[2] Recently, the big three automakers have been pushing their liability for health costs onto their unions, replacing their previous guarantee of full employee and retiree health coverage with lump sum payments to establish (underfunded) union-run health care trust funds.

Meanwhile, low-wage employers like Wal-Mart gain competitive advantage by purchasing goods made overseas (where health benefit costs are low) and offering only the skimpiest of health coverage to their US workers. Governments face a double whammy: burgeoning benefit costs for their public employees (eg, teachers, firemen, police) and sharply escalating costs for public programs, such as Medicaid and Medicare.

As employers attempt to shed the costs of health care, working families increasingly find care and coverage unaffordable. In 2005, 18% of middle-income adults lacked health insurance for at least part of the year, up from 13% in 2001.[3] Nearly a quarter of Americans report being unable to pay medical bills, and 13% had been contacted by a collection agency about a medical bill within the past year.[3] Eighteen percent of those with coverage (and 43% of the uninsured) failed to fill a prescription last year because of cost, and millions forego routine preventive care, such as Papanicolaou smears, mammograms, and colon cancer screening, because of lack of coverage.[3] More than half of American families in bankruptcy courts are there, at least in part, because of medical illness or medical bills, and three quarters of the medically bankrupt had health insurance at the onset of the illness that bankrupted them.[4]

The authors advocate a fundamental change in health care financing—national health insurance (NHI)—because lesser measures, such as Medicaid expansions and government mandates that people buy private insurance, have been tried and failed. Moreover, the alternative to NHI advocated by the Bush administration—so-called consumer-directed health care (CDH)—would actually make matters worse. As discussed in detail elsewhere in this article, CDH would financially penalize older and sicker patients, deter millions from seeking needed care, shift additional medical resources to those who are already well served,

Harvard Medical School, Department of Medicine, Cambridge Hospital, 1493 Cambridge Street, Cambridge MA 02139, USA

* Corresponding author.

E-mail address: steffie_woolhandler@hms.harvard.edu (S. Woolhandler).

Urol Clin N Am 36 (2009) 57–62
doi:10.1016/j.ucl.2008.08.007

further inflate bureaucracy, and do little or nothing to contain costs.

FAILURE OF INCREMENTAL REFORMS

Since the implementation of Medicare and Medicaid in the late 1960s, a welter of piecemeal reforms have aimed to reduce medical costs and expand coverage. Health maintenance organizations (HMOs) and diagnosis-related groups (DRGs) promised to moderate health spending and free up funds to expand coverage. Tens of billions have been allocated to expanding Medicaid and similar programs for children. Medicare and Medicaid have tried managed care. Tennessee promised nearly universal coverage under the TennCare program, and several states have implemented high-risk pools to insure high-cost individuals. For-profit firms, which allege that they bring business-like efficiency to health care, now own most HMOs, dialysis clinics, and nursing homes, in addition to many hospitals, and in accordance with the prescription of many economists, the health care marketplace has become increasingly competitive. Yet, none of these initiatives have put a brake on the relentless increases in the number of uninsured, the soaring costs of care, or the rising number and power of health care bureaucrats.

Mandate Model Reforms

The experience of three states with incremental reforms deserves particular attention, because each tried to achieve universal health care using a "mandate model" (sometimes called "mixed model"), now advocated by leading Democrats. Such reforms couple an expansion of Medicaid (or a similar public program) with a mandate that people (or their employers) purchase private insurance coverage. This model was first proposed by Richard Nixon in 1971 and was first enacted into law in 1988 by Massachusetts Governor Michael Dukakis on the eve of his presidential bid.

The Dukakis plan levied a fine on employers who failed to purchase private coverage for their employees and included an individual mandate requiring self-employed persons and adult students to purchase their own unsubsidized coverage. In 1989, Oregon passed a similar mandate-model reform (with expanded Medicaid eligibility and an employer mandate). The Oregon plan also included a highly publicized provision rationing expensive services, such as bone marrow transplants, for Medicaid recipients. Washington State followed, with the passage of another mandate model reform (which included an individual mandate similar to the one in the Dukakis plan) in 1993.

In all three cases, politicians and major media outlets, such as the New York Times, trumpeted the new laws as achieving universal coverage. In all cases, it soon became evident that the costs of the new coverage were unsustainable and the laws died quiet deaths. State legislators backed away from enforcing the mandates and eventually repealed them. Even when legislators found funds to expand Medicaid, gains in coverage were offset by the continued erosion of employer-sponsored insurance. None of the three states saw a drop in the numbers of uninsured residents, even in the short term.

The latest iteration of mandate model reform was passed in 2006 by Massachusetts Governor Mitt Romney and the Democratically controlled state legislature. As in the earlier reforms, Massachusetts' 2006 law expanded Medicaid, offered subsidized Medicaid-like coverage for the near poor, and imposed a fine on employers failing to cover their workers, although the 2006 law's employer fine is quite modest (at most, $295 per worker annually). The novel feature of the new law is its extensive and punitive "individual mandate"—a requirement that hundreds of thousands of middle-income uninsured persons buy their own coverage. For a 56-year-old single man earning $31,000 (ie, more than 300% of poverty), the cheapest available plan costs $4100 and comes with a $2000 deductible that must be met before his providers collect anything from insurance. When the full fines kick in at the end of 2008, he could be fined $982 annually if he refuses to buy the policy. Yet, such skimpy coverage might leave him worse off than no coverage at all; illness would still bring crippling out-of-pocket costs, but the $4100 annual premium would have emptied his bank account even before the bills start arriving. Little wonder that among those required to buy such unsubsidized coverage, only 4% had signed up as of November 1, 2007. Meanwhile, the state just announced a $147 million funding shortfall, threatening the subsidized coverage for the poor.[5]

The 2006 Massachusetts reform, like all such patchwork reforms, is already foundering on a simple problem: expanding coverage must increase costs unless resources are diverted from elsewhere in the system. With US health costs nearly double those of any other nation and rising more rapidly[6] and government budgets already stretched, large infusions of new money are unlikely to be sustainable.

Without new money, patchwork reforms can only expand coverage by siphoning resources from clinical care. Advocates of managed care and market competition once argued that their strategy could accomplish this by trimming clinical fat. Unfortunately, new layers of bureaucrats have invariably overseen the managed care "diet" prescribed for clinicians and patients. Such cost management bureaucracies have proved not only intrusive but expensive, devouring any clinical savings. For instance, HMOs in the Medicare program now cost the taxpayers at least 12% more per enrollee than the costs of caring for similar patients under traditional Medicare.[7]

Resources seep inexorably from the bedside to administrative offices. The shortage of bedside nurses coincides with the growing number of registered nurse utilization reviewers. Productivity pressures mount for clinicians, whereas colleagues who have moved from the bedside to the executive suite rule our profession. Bureaucracy now consumes nearly a third of our health care budget.[8]

CONSUMER-DIRECTED HEALTH CARE, ANOTHER DISAPPOINTMENT

A popular policy nostrum, CDH, is premised on the idea that Americans are too well insured, painting them as voracious medical consumers too insulated from the costs of their care. CDH proponents advocate sharply higher insurance deductibles (eg, $5000 for an individual or $10,000 for a family) as the stimulus needed to make Americans wiser medical consumers. In policy wonks' dreams, these high-deductible policies are coupled with health savings accounts (HSAs), which are tax-free accounts that can be used to pay the deductible and medical services, such as cosmetic surgery, that are entirely excluded from coverage. In practice, however, most employees covered by CDH plans receive little or no employer contribution to their HSA,[9] leaving many patients at risk for massive uncovered bills without savings with which to pay them.

CDH plans may benefit those who are young, healthy, and wealthy but threaten the old, sick, and poor. Under CDH, those with low medical expenses win; they get lower premiums, pay trivial out-of-pocket expenses, and perhaps accumulate some tax-advantaged savings in their HSA. Patients needing care lose, however. For instance, virtually anyone with diabetes or heart disease is sure to pay more under CDH plans. For them, the higher out-of-pocket costs required before coverage kicks in exceed any premium savings. Even those with only hypercholesterolemia or hypertension face higher costs unless they forego needed medications or other care.

CDH incentives selectively discourage low-cost primary and preventive care, although doing nothing to reduce the high-cost care that accounts for most health spending. High deductibles cause many to think twice before opting for a routine mammogram, prostate-specific antigen (PSA) screening, cholesterol check, or colonoscopy. In the Rand Health Insurance Experiment, the only randomized trial of such health insurance arrangements, high deductible policies caused a 17% decline in toddler immunizations, a 19% drop in Papanicolaou tests, and a 30% decrease in preventive care for men.[10] Although high deductibles caused a 30% drop in visits for minor symptoms, they also resulted in a 20% decline in visits for serious symptoms, such as loss of consciousness or exercised-induced chest pain.[10] Most patients have no way of knowing whether their chest discomfort signals indigestion or ischemia.

Although CDH discourages many patients from seeking routine low-cost care, those with severe acute illnesses have no choice. Even 1 day in the hospital pushes most patients past CDH plans' high-deductible thresholds, leaving the patient with a large bill for the first day of care but with no further incentive to be a prudent purchaser. Hence, CDH incentives inflict financial pain on the severely ill, who account for 80% of all health costs, but have little impact on the overall costs of their care.

Moreover, the risk-selection incentives inherent in CDH threaten to raise the cost of other insurance options. As younger and healthier (ie, lower cost) patients shift to CDH plans, premiums for the sick who remain in non-CDH coverage are going to skyrocket. Already in the Federal Employee Health Benefits Program, CDH plans are segregating young men from the costlier female and older workers.[11] According to a leaked memo, Wal-Mart's board of directors considered offering CDH plans to its employees as an explicit strategy to push sicker high-cost workers to quit.[12]

CDH also seems unfair on other accounts. The tax breaks for HSAs selectively reward the wealthiest Americans. A single father who makes $16,000 annually would save $19.60 in income taxes by putting $2000 into an HSA.[13] A similar father earning $450,000 would save $720 in taxes.

If making Americans pay more out of their pockets for care could constrain health care costs, it would already have done so; the United States already has the world's highest out-of-pocket costs for care and the highest health costs. Copayments in Switzerland, a nation near the top of the charts in health spending, have not reduced total health expenditures.[14] In Canada, charging copayments had little impact on costs; doctors less frequently saw the poor (and often sick) patients who could not pay but filled their appointment slots with more affluent patients who could.[15,16] Higher copayments for medications in Quebec resulted in increased emergency department (ED) visits, hospitalizations, and deaths for the poor and elderly.[17] Similarly, capping drug coverage for Medicare beneficiaries in the Kaiser HMO caused a sharp drop in adherence to drug therapy (in addition to an increase in lipids, blood pressure, and blood glucose) but no change in overall health costs.[18]

Moreover, CDH and HSAs add new layers of expensive health care bureaucracy. Already, insurers and investment firms are vying for the estimated $1 billion annually in fees for managing HSAs.[19] CDH would force physicians to collect fees directly from patients (many of them unable to pay), a task that is even costlier than billing insurers,[20] while still making us play by insurers' utilization review and documentation rules; failure to do so disqualifies bills from counting toward the patient's deductible.

Although CDH proponents paint a rosy picture of consumer responsiveness and personal responsibility, CDH would punish the sick and middle aged while rewarding the healthy and young. Employees would bear more of the burden, and employers would bear less. Working families would be forced to skimp on vital care, whereas the rich would enjoy tax-free tummy tucks. In addition, as in every health reform in memory, bureaucrats and insurance firms would walk off with an ever larger share of health dollars.

The Case for National Health Insurance

In contrast to CDH, a properly structured NHI program could expand coverage without increasing costs by reducing the huge health administrative apparatus that now consumes 31% of total health spending. Health care's enormous bureaucratic burden is a peculiarly American phenomenon. No nation with NHI spends even half as much administering care or tolerates the bureaucratic intrusions in clinical care that have become routine in the United States. Indeed, administrative overhead in Canada's health system, which resembles that of the United States in its emphasis on private fee-for-service–based practice, is approximately half of the US level.[8]

Our biggest HMOs keep 20%, even 25%, of premiums for their overhead and profit;[21] Canada's NHI has 1% overhead, and even US Medicare takes less than 4%.[8,22] In addition, HMOs inflict mountains of paperwork on doctors and hospitals. The average US hospital spends one quarter of its budget on billing and administration, nearly twice the average in Canada. American physicians spend nearly 8 hours per week on paperwork, and employ 1.66 clerical workers per doctor,[23] far more than in Canada.[8]

Reducing our bureaucratic apparatus to Canadian levels would save approximately 15% of current health spending, $340 billion annually, enough to cover the uninsured fully and to upgrade coverage for those who are now underinsured. Proponents of NHI,[24] disinterested civil servants,[25,26] and even skeptics[27] all agree on this point.

Unfortunately, neither piecemeal tinkering nor wholesale computerization[28] can achieve significant bureaucratic savings. The key to administrative simplicity in Canada (and other nations) is single-source payment. Canadian hospitals (mostly private nonprofit institutions) are paid a global annual budget to cover all costs, much as a fire department is funded in the United States, obviating the need for administratively complex per-patient billing. Canadian physicians (most of whom are in private practice) bill by checking a box on a simple insurance form. Fee schedules are negotiated annually between provincial medical associations and governments. All patients have the same coverage.

Unfortunately, during the 1990s, Canada's program was starved of funds by a federal government that faced budget deficits, reflecting the pressure from the wealthy to avoid paying taxes to cross-subsidize care (and other services) for the sick and poor. Whereas Canadian and US health spending was once comparable, today, Canada spends barely half (per capita) what we do.[6] Shortages of a few types of expensive high-technology care have resulted.

Nevertheless, Canada's health outcomes remain better than ours (eg, life expectancy is 2 years longer), and most quality comparisons indicate that Canadians enjoy care at least equivalent to that for insured Americans.[6,29] Moreover, the extent of shortages and waiting lists has been greatly exaggerated.

In British Columbia, the provincial Ministry of Health posts current surgical waiting times,[30] making it is possible to follow surgical waiting lists in real time. Information on waits for urologic surgery is available.[31] As of the middle of October 2007, at the highest volume urologic surgery center (Greater Victoria Hospital), 1 of the 7 urologists had no wait for a "priority 1" surgical patient. Three other surgeons listed expected waits of 1 or 2 weeks. The surgeons' wait times for lower priority cases range from 0 to 10 weeks. At the second most active urologic center, none of the 10 urologists report a wait for priority 1 patients. Lower priority patients can expect a median wait of 4 weeks, but actual waits vary depending on their choice of surgeon. It seems unlikely that waits of this magnitude constitute an important health hazard. A system structured like Canada's but with nearly double the funding (ie, the current level of health funding available in the United States) could deliver high-quality care without the modest waits or shortages that Canadians have experienced.

The NHI that the authors and many colleagues have proposed would create a single tax-funded comprehensive insurer in each state, federally mandated but locally controlled.[32] Everyone would be fully insured for all medically necessary services, and private insurance duplicating the NHI coverage would be proscribed (as is currently the case with Medicare). The current Byzantine insurance bureaucracy with its tangle of regulations and duplicative paperwork would be dismantled. Instead, the NHI trust fund would dispense all payments, and central administrative costs would be limited by law to less than 3% of total health spending.

The NHI would negotiate an annual global budget with each hospital based on past expenditures, projected changes in costs and use, and proposed new and innovative programs. Many hospital administrative tasks would disappear. Hospitals would have no bills to keep track of, no eligibility determination, and no need to attribute costs and charges to individual patients.

Group practices and clinics could elect to be paid fees for service or receive global budgets similar to hospitals. Although HMOs that merely contract with outside providers for care would be eliminated, those that actually employ physicians and own clinical facilities could receive global budgets, fees for service, or capitation payments (with the proviso that capitation payments could not be diverted to profits or exorbitant executive compensation). As in Canada, physicians could elect to be paid on a fee-for-service basis or could receive salaries from hospitals, clinics, or HMOs.

A sound NHI program would not raise costs; administrative savings would pay for the expanded coverage. Although NHI would require new taxes, these would be fully offset by a decrease in insurance premiums and out-of-pocket costs. Moreover, the additional tax burden would be smaller than is usually appreciated, because nearly 60% of health spending is already tax supported (versus roughly 70% in Canada).[33] In addition to Medicare, Medicaid, and other explicit public programs, our governments fund tax subsidies for private insurance, costing the federal government alone more than $188 billion annually.[34] In addition, local, state, and federal agencies that purchase private coverage for government workers account for 24.2% of total employer health insurance spending,[35] dollars that should properly be viewed as a public rather than a private health expenditure.

The NHI that the authors propose faces important political obstacles. Private insurance firms and HMOs staunchly oppose NHI, which would eliminate them along with the 8-, 9-, and even 10-figure incomes of their executives. Similarly, investor-owned hospitals and drug firms fear that NHI would curtail their profits. The pharmaceutical industry rightly fears that an NHI system would bargain for lower drug prices, as has occurred in other nations.

Practical problems in implementing NHI also loom. The financial viability of the system that the authors propose depends on achieving and maintaining administrative simplicity. The single-payer macromanagement approach to cost control (which relies on readily enforceable overall budgetary limits) is inherently less administratively complex than our current micromanagement approach, with its case-by-case scrutiny of billions of individual expenditures and encounters. Even under NHI, however, vigilance (and statutory limits) would be needed to curb the tendency of bureaucracy to reproduce and amplify itself.

NHI would reorient the way we pay for care, bringing the hundreds of billions now squandered on malignant bureaucracy back to the bedside. NHI could restore the physician-patient relationship, offer patients a free choice of physicians and hospitals, and free physicians from the hassles of insurance paperwork.

Patchwork reforms cannot simultaneously address the twin problems of cost and access. CDH is a thinly veiled program to cut back on already threadbare insurance coverage and offers no real hope of cost containment. NHI offers the only viable option for health care reform. The authors invite colleagues to join with the 14,000 members of Physicians for a National Health Program [36] in advocating for such reform.

REFERENCES

1. Institute of Medicine. Insuring America's health: principles and recommendations. Washington, DC: National Academies Press; 2004.
2. Taylor M. Applying the brakes. Mod Healthc 2005; 35(43):14.
3. Collins SR, Davis K, Doty MM, et al. Gaps in health insurance: an all-American problem. Findings from the Common wealth Fund biennial health insurance survey. New York: Commonwealth Fund; 2006.
4. Himmelstein DU, Warren E, Thorne D, et al. Illness and injury as contributors to bankruptcy. Health Aff–Web Exclusive; 2005.
5. Dembner A. Success could put health plan in the red. Boston Globe (November 18, 2007) Available at: http://www.boston.com/news/local/articles/2007/

11/18/success_could_put_health_plan_in_the_red/. Accessed November 20, 2007.

6. Organization for Economic Cooperation and Development (OECD). OECD health data 2005. Computer database (Paris. OECD, 2005).

7. Miller (Executive Director, MEDPAC) ME. The Medicare Advantage program. Testimony before the Committee on the Budget, U.S. House of Representatives. Available at: http://www.medpac.gov/documents/062807_Housebudget_MedPAC_testimony_MA.pdf 2007. Accessed October 12, 2007.

8. Woolhandler S, Campbell T, Himmelstein DU. Health care administration costs in the U.S. and Canada. N Engl J Med 2003;349:768–75.

9. EBRI/Commonwealth Fund Survey. Available at: http://www.ebri.org/publications/ib/index.cfm?fa=ibDisp&content_id=3769. 2006. Accessed October 30, 2007.

10. Newhouse JP and the Insurance Experiment Group. Free for all? Lessons from the Rand Health Insurance Experiment. Cambridge (MA): Harvard University Press; 1993.

11. United States Government Accountability Office. Federal Employees Health Benefits Program: early experience with consumer-directed health plans. Washington, DC: November 2005. GAO-06-143. Available at: http://www.gao.gov/new.items/d06143.pdf. Accessed February 14, 2006.

12. Supplemental benefits documentation: Board of Directors Retreat FY06 Wal-Mart Stores, Inc. Available at: http://www.nytimes.com/packages/pdf/business/26walmart.pdf. Accessed February 14, 2006.

13. Tax Policy Center. Effective marginal federal income tax rates for a head of household with one child in 2005. Available at: http://www.taxpolicycenter.org/TaxFacts/TFDB/Content/Excel/effective_marginal_hoh1_2005.xls. Accessed February 14, 2006.

14. Conference Board of Canada. Challenging health care system sustainability, understanding health system performance of leading countries. Available at: http://www.conferenceboard.ca/boardwiseii/signin.asp. 2004. Accessed October 2007.

15. Enterline PE, Salter V, McDonald AD, et al. The distribution of medical services before and after "free" medical care—the Quebec experience. N Engl J Med 1973;289(22):1174–8.

16. Beck RG, Horne JM. Utilization of publicly insured health services in Saskatchewan before, during and after copayment. Med Care 1980;18(8):787–806.

17. Tamblyn R, Laprise R, Hanley JA, et al. Adverse events associated with prescription drug cost-sharing among poor and elderly persons. JAMA 2001;285(4):421–9.

18. Hsu J, Price M, Huang J, et al. Unintended consequences of caps on Medicare drug benefits. N Engl J Med 2006;354:2349–59.

19. Becker C. One question: credit or debit? As health savings accounts gain in popularity, insurers and the financial services industry want to bank the cash. Mod Healthc 2006;6–16.

20. Romano M. Driven to distress. Mod Healthc 2006;28–30.

21. Special report. BestWeek Life/Health. April 12, 1999.

22. Heffler S, Levit K, Smith S, et al. Health spending growth up in 1999; faster growth expected in the future. Health Aff 2001;20(2):193–203.

23. Remler DK, Gray BM, Newhouse JP. Does managed care mean more hassles for physicians? Inquiry 2000;37:304–16.

24. Grumbach K, Bodenheimer T, Woolhandler S, et al. Liberal benefits conservative spending: the Physicians for a National Health Program proposal. JAMA 1991;265:2549–54.

25. U.S. General Accounting Office. Canadian health insurance: lessons for the United States. Washington, DC: U.S. Government Printing Office; 1991. (GAO/HRD-91-90).

26. Congress of the United States Congressional Budget Office. Universal health insurance coverage using Medicare's payment rates. Washington, DC: U.S. Government Printing Office; 1991.

27. Sheils JF, Haught RA. Analysis of the costs and impact of universal health care coverage under a single payer model for the state of Vermont. The Lewin Group Inc.; 2001.

28. Himmelstein DU, Woolhandler S. Hope and hype: predicting the impact of electronic medical records. Health Aff 2005;24(5):1121–3.

29. Lasser KE, Himmelstein DU, Woolhandler S. Access to care, health status, and health disparities in the United States and Canada: results of a cross-national population-based survey. Am J Public Health 2006;96:1300–7.

30. Available at: http://www.hlth.gov.bc.ca/waitlist/.html.

31. Available at: http://www.swl.hlth.gov.bc.ca/swl/swl_db/swl.WaitlistPkg.GetHospitalListBySurgSpecNLF?lEvent=UR.

32. Woolhandler S, Himmelstein DU, Angell M, et al. Proposal of the Physicians' Working Group for Single-Payer National Health Insurance. JAMA 2003;290:798–805.

33. Woolhandler S, Himmelstein DU. Paying for national health insurance—and not getting it: taxes pay for a larger share of U.S. health care than most Americans think they do. Health Aff 2002; 21(4):88–98.

34. Sheils J, Haught R. The cost of tax-exempt health benefits in 2004. Health Aff Web Exclusive Posted. Available at: http://content.healthaffairs.org/cgi/reprint/hlthaff.w4.106v1; 2004. Accessed June 6, 2006.

35. Office of the Actuary. National Center for Health Statistics. Sponsors of health care costs: businesses, households and governments. 1987–2004. Available at: http://www.cms.hhs.gov/NationalHealthExpendData/downloads/bhg06.pdf. Accessed June 6, 2006.

36. Available at: www.PNHP.org.

The American Medical Association Stake in the Future of US Health Care: The American Medical Association Plan for Reform of the US Health Care System

William G. Plested III, MD

KEYWORDS

- American Medical Association • Ownership
- Tax reform • Individual responsibility
- Insurance reform • Facilitating market innovation
- Antitrust reform • Medical liability reform

This article discusses the most important thing in one's life: health and the health of one's families and loved ones.

To fully understand and appreciate where society is today, the author finds it useful to recall his own childhood in Wichita, Kansas. Summertime in Wichita is hot. Not hot like Las Vegas or Death Valley, but hot like 100 to 110°, with, 90-plus percent humidity. Hot that oppressive makes the air feel like one is breathing split pea soup through a swizzle stick. What was available was a huge municipal swimming pool that was understandably a favorite of kids of all ages.

The author was able to enjoy a refreshing afternoon in the pool a couple of times, but then suddenly his mother would not allow him to go anymore. He was devastated, but her decision was not punishment. It was an act of fear and an act of love, because in those days, there was a horrible disease that afflicted people of all ages, but especially children. No one was safe. Not even the president of the United States could escape its debilitating grasp.[1] The author will never know if staying away from hundreds of kids in that municipal pool made a difference, but he was one of the lucky children not to be stricken. Later, in

medical school, however, the author took care of children in Drinker respirators. Today, many medical students have not heard of a Drinker, and certainly have not taken care of a patient using one. A Drinker respirator was known commonly as an iron lung.[2] Nothing is more striking than a terrified, completely helpless child encased in an iron lung.

That all changed overnight with Salk's discovery of a vaccine.[3] Because of this medical miracle, children and their parents no longer live in deathly fear of this crippling and lethal disease.

But a vaccine to prevent polio is only the tip of a huge iceberg of medical progress. If one looks back only a short time, the medical textbooks and conferences did not mention the diagnostic prowess of CT scans, positron emission tomography (PET) scans, MRIs, ultrasounds, Doppler, and angiograms, because they simply did not exist. There were no heart–lung machines, artificial vessels, valves, pacemakers, defibrillators, or stents. Major surgery always involved big incisions. Video-assisted endoscopic procedures and robotics were science fiction rather than routine care.

The point is that health care technology in those days surrounding World War II was precious little,

American Medical Association, 515 North State Street, Chicago, IL 60610, USA
E-mail address: william_plested@mam_assn.org

Urol Clin N Am 36 (2009) 63–71
doi:10.1016/j.ucl.2008.08.012

and physicians knew it. Yet, that great generation of physicians did what now is so rare that it seems quaint. Physicians made house calls. They cared for entire families. They did what doctors have done for centuries; they were there when it mattered, with whatever technology was available, but more importantly with caring and compassion. Patients appreciated that care, and still do today.

But something happened along the way, the endless onslaught of medical advances inevitably was accompanied by costs that rose to staggering levels, levels that became beyond the reach of many patients. Government and insurers leaped into action with promises of solutions. But they did so by insinuating themselves into the patient–physician relationship. Their promise, continued to this very day, is to "provide the best care at the lowest price." That primrose promise prompted a heap of rules, regulations, and red tape that have been foisted upon physicians' backs. To accomplish the goal of reduced costs, both government and insurers systematically have enacted changes designed to exercise complete control over physicians (ie, training, daily practices, what they order, what they recommend, and what they are paid). Today these infringements have become like the Medusa; one noxious serpent is cut off, only to have two others sprout up.

The result of all of these schemes has been a hodgepodge of medical care directed by a mind-numbing array of rules, and an overworked and discouraged physician workforce whose reimbursement in many cases does not even cover the costs of delivering care. In addition, the ranks of those who cannot afford care or health insurance have increased year after year.

One now hears increasingly strident cries of a "health care crisis." The author wants to emphasize that this is not a medical crisis, because history shows not medical failure but an unprecedented record of medical progress and success. Because of medical progress, people now live much longer and with less disability than ever before. If, in fact, there is a crisis, it is not a medical crisis, but a crisis about who will pay—for the incredible medical care that today is taken for granted.

Inevitably, when costs become beyond the grasp of most people, there are calls for the government to step in and pay the bills. Such calls are heard on a daily basis. Government meddling, however, becomes more and more inadequate as the complexity of the issue at hand increases. And nothing is more complicated than modern medicine.

Government has only two extremely blunt instruments in its armamentarium: wage and price controls, and rationing. All government schemes to change health care consist of a variety of these two instruments, and neither work, primarily because government refuses to be honest with the public about what it really is doing. Instead of saying that there are real limits, promises of the best care at the lowest price continue to be the mantra.

The time for rose-colored glasses, meaningless promises, and half-hearted measures has past. The American Medical Association (AMA) has—for more than a decade—urged the conscience of America to act. The AMA, comprised of physicians of all ages and all specialties, cannot do it alone, which is why physicians are taking their national call for America to America.

Recently, the AMA launched the Voice for the Uninsured Campaign,[4] a multiyear effort designed to promote awareness, spur voters to action, and culminate with the passage of legislation to bring real reform to the health care delivery system. The AMA plan will expand coverage for the uninsured, increase access to care, and make certain that all Americans have access to medical insurance. Of equal importance is that the AMA plans to make certain that those who now are insured will not lose their insurance if they become ill, if they move, change jobs, or are laid off.

Over the next year, the AMA will be on the campaign trail—not with any one candidate—but with all of them, and with patients and community leaders in the chambers of commerce, rotary clubs, lions clubs, economic roundtables, and anywhere and everywhere else physicians can visit.

The reason is simple; in addition to the 47 million uninsured[5]—one in seven Americans—and the vast majority of Americans who are insured and fear losing that insurance, need physicians to step up and make a difference. Why does the author think that this can succeed? Simply because unlike government, insurers, and employers, physicians have the most potent instrument in their medical bags, their patients' trust.[6]

In the coming year, physicians need to harness that trust and urge their patients to demand action from the candidates. Not just the ones parading on CNN, but the ones patients meet with at their local town hall. Call them up. Tell them that next November—when patients go into that voting booth, there need to be three simple questions in the front of their minds:

1. Where do the candidates stand on the health care issues facing the nation?
2. What are they going to do about it?
3. Will they support and enact the AMA plan for reform?

The debate today is not about whether all Americans should have health insurance and access to a physician, but how to get there.

WHO ARE THE UNINSURED?

The US Census Bureau tells that there are 47 million uninsured Americans (ie, 47 million Americans who in general are living sicker and dying younger than those with health insurance).[7] According to the Institute of Medicine, a lack of coverage costs 18 thousand needless deaths a year.[8] Yet four out of five uninsured are in families that have at least one employed person.[9]

Being uninsured produces a level of stress and insecurity like few other life circumstances. And everyone pays. The United States spends nearly $100 billion annually to provide health services to uninsured patients.[10] And each year, physicians routinely contribute $20 billion in charity care. They also write off another $20 billion as bad debt. This is inefficient, inconsistent, and inexcusable.

Why is this happening? Between 2001 and 2007, premiums for employer-sponsored health insurance increased 78%;[11] in 6 years, the author doubts physician income increased 78%. Employers able to offer health insurance decreased from 69% in 2000 to 60% in 2007.[11] Fewer than half (45%) of small-sized businesses (three to nine workers) offer health insurance.[11] To put it simply, they cannot offer what they cannot afford.

Given these staggering numbers, the AMA has come to the conclusion that the candidates' back and forth of sound bites and warring policy theories need to be replaced by concrete steps and definitive action.

For that to happen, voters must demand that their candidates have a plan, and voters must keep that plan in mind when they decide who their candidate will be. Patients want their physician's best diagnosis and treatment. The AMA wants candidates to make certain that they also go to the nations' doctors to get the best treatment plan. This is not a choice that can wait much longer.

HOW DID WE GET HERE?

The employment-based medical insurance system arose out of the wage and price controls that were imposed by the government during World War II. This was done in an attempt to prevent rapid escalation of manufacturing costs related to the war effort. Also, government allowed employers to offer health insurance and other nonwage benefits in lieu of wage increases. Employers thus could use offerings of these benefits to attract employees, who were in high demand during the war.[12] Subsequently, the Internal Revenue Service

(IRS) ruled that employer costs for employee health insurance could be excluded from taxable compensation for the employee.[13] That IRS ruling still stands, although it is obsolete for today's population, because it has had the pervasive consequence of encouraging job lock, which keeps people in their jobs because they cannot obtain health insurance on their own or may not be able to when they switch jobs. Job lock is squarely at odds with today's more mobile and flexible workforce.

As is evident, today's workers are extremely mobile. This, in the system of employment-based health insurance, means that coverage changes often. This is complicated by the fact that like others, employers did not anticipate the rise in health care costs. This reality became apparent decades after employment-based coverage had become an entrenched worker expectation. Old bargaining agreements that covered everything medicine had to offer were based on the days mentioned previously, when everything was precious little.

WHAT DOES THE AMERICAN MEDICAL ASSOCIATION THINK NEEDS TO BE DONE?

To this day, the government continues to subsidize the purchase of health insurance by excluding expenditures on health insurance from an individual's or family's taxable income, but only if insurance is obtained through an employer.[14] Usually that includes only that portion of the premium paid for by the employer. It makes little sense that the self-employed can deduct 100% of their insurance costs while no tax break is given to individuals who purchase their own health insurance, or to workers whose employers do not offer coverage.

The AMA has represented America's physicians since 1847, and it has been involved directly with patients and health care policy ever since. The AMA's experience and research give it insight on starting toward a solution. The AMA can and should take the lead in informing every American and every potential political leader about its plan to ease the burden.

AMA members have studied and visited countries with different health care systems around the world. It is crystal clear that today, no country and no system in the world are immune to the problems of rising costs, increasing and aging populations, and a concomitant lack of political wisdom and will. The twin tsunamis of technology and demography do not respect national boundaries. Everybody seems to have an answer, but these answers are usually little more than a simple list of laudable goals. Invariably, the means to achieve those goals often wither under close scrutiny. Legislators routinely meet their Waterloo when they attempt to fund these Utopian plans.[15] This is why the AMA plan is based on clearly articulated principles that should be used for anyone who wishes to develop a plan to reform the health insurance system. The main elements of our plan are: individual ownership, tax reform, insurance reforms, and medical liability reform.

Ownership

The centerpiece of the AMA plan is that each person must own his or her personal health insurance policy. It makes absolutely no sense for an employer, the government, or any other outside party to claim this ownership. Individual ownership means that the policy will stay with the patient. This guarantees portability. Each person can, and should be able to purchase a health insurance plan that fits his or her specific needs. Next, ownership must be separated from payment. If an employer decides to cover all or part of the premium, that is acceptable, but the employer would not own the policy. For those who, for whatever reason, cannot afford coverage, the government would provide assistance through tax credits or vouchers that could be used only for the purchase of health insurance, but government also must not own the policy.

Tax Reform

The current tax treatment of employment-based health insurance also needs overhaul. As noted previously, under the current system, an employer's expenditures on health insurance are not considered to be taxable income to the employee. There are no similar tax benefits for anyone who does not receive insurance through an employer. This inequity should be replaced with refundable and advance-able tax credits that apply to all individuals who purchase health insurance.

Under the AMA's proposed system, employer contributions to health insurance would be reported as taxable compensation. Individuals would be given health insurance tax credits that would be subtracted from their directly from their tax bills. All others would similarly be able to apply for a tax credit arising from their expenditures for health care insurance. The AMA believes that expanding health insurance coverage through the use of tax credits should be guided by the following principles:

The size of tax credits should be related inversely to income. Those who have lower incomes of necessity need greater subsidies than those who have higher incomes. Targeting subsidies toward those who otherwise most likely would be uninsured conserves budgetary resources. Tax credits should be contingent on the purchase of health insurance, so that if insurance is not obtained, the credit is not provided. This principle provides a strong incentive for people to obtain health insurance voluntarily. Individuals and families could receive tax credits whether they obtain their health insurance through employment or elsewhere.

Tax credits should be refundable. This means that those who have low incomes would receive a check or voucher from the government to be used only for purchasing health insurance, and this would apply when they owe less in taxes than the value of the tax credit. Those who have higher incomes would use their tax credits to offset their tax liability.

Tax credits or vouchers should be available in advance for those who have low incomes. Tax credits should be advance-able so that those who have low incomes, and those who cannot afford the monthly out-of-pocket premium costs, would be able to purchase coverage without waiting for the year-end tax reconciliation process.

The size of tax credits should be large enough to ensure that health insurance is affordable for most people. Tax credits need to be large enough to empower virtually all individuals to obtain and maintain a basic health insurance plan. At the lowest income levels, the credit must approach 100% of the premium.

The size of tax credits should vary with family size to mirror the pricing structure of insurance premiums. In general, tax credits should mirror the pricing structure of health insurance premiums for individuals and families, with premiums for family policies being less than the sum of premiums for individual members.

Tax credits should be fixed-dollar amounts for a given income and family structure. To encourage individuals to be cost-conscious and to discourage overinsurance, the size of credits should be independent of the actual cost of the plan chosen by the patient.

The size of tax credits should be capped in any given year. The preceding principle calls for tax credits to be fixed-dollar amounts. If tax credits nevertheless are designed to vary with the price of insurance, the credits should be capped to prevent overnment-subsidized overinsurance.

Tax credits for families should be contingent on each member of the family having health insurance. In the absence of this requirement, individuals might game the system by purchasing coverage only for themselves and not their healthy children, waiting to seek coverage for the children only when they experience a need for health care. This principle ensures maximum coverage.

Tax credits should be applicable only for the purchase of health insurance, and not for out-of-pocket health expenditures. This principle limits the tax credits to the purchase of health insurance coverage, including health savings accounts. Allowing tax credits to be used for an unlimited array of out-of-pocket expenses could encourage inappropriate use of health services.

A system of income-related, refundable tax credits come close to providing health care coverage for all Americans, particularly once a mechanism is in place to give the refundable credit in advance to those who earn too little to pay income tax.

The AMA tax credit approach is a targeted and incremental approach. The AMA believes tax credits that must be used to purchase private insurance are preferable to public sector expansions as a means of providing coverage to the uninsured. Because AMA members pragmatically recognize there are finite resources, the AMA supports implementing individual tax credits for the purchase of health insurance for specific target populations such as low-income workers, low-income individuals, children, and the chronically ill.

In addition, the AMA also supports innovative state-based demonstration projects, including, but not limited to, implementing income-related, refundable, and advance-able tax credits.

Individual Responsibility

The AMA plan supports individual responsibility. AMA members believe in the strengths of the free market, not in a free lunch. Currently, everyone pays inflated premiums because of the costs associated with treating the uninsured, and these inflated premium rates constitute an additional barrier to coverage, not only for the uninsured, but for those who accept the responsibility to provide coverage for themselves and their families.

The AMA supports requiring individuals and families earning greater than 500% percent of the federal poverty level (FPL) ($51,050 for individuals and $103,250 for a family of four) to obtain, at a minimum, coverage for catastrophic health care and evidence-based preventive health care—a basic health care policy. There should be tax implications for noncompliance. Those who conscientiously provide for themselves and their dependents should not be penalized by the potentially costly medical treatments of those who have the ability to purchase health insurance coverage but remain uninsured. It is important to recognize that individual responsibility with tax implications for noncompliance is distinct from an individual mandate, which implies that the failure to obtain coverage could result in criminal penalties.

Most of the uninsured (89%) have incomes below 500% of the FPL. AMA support for requiring that these individuals and families obtain coverage is contingent upon implementation of a system of refundable tax credits or other subsidies. All the pieces must fit together in a coherent whole rather than a politically popular, but practically unworkable proposal that may garner applause lines now but later languish as yet another platitude to earn votes rather than drive honest reform and true coverage.

Insurance Reform

Patients should be able choose their own doctor, their own hospital, and the insurance coverage that meets their specific needs and that they can afford. The AMA believes that a working health system enables individuals not only to own and but to also be able to choose their health insurance plan. Currently, only one in six companies that now offer health insurance offers their employees a choice of plans. Under the AMA proposal, individuals, rather than employers, would choose the kind of coverage they want, whether through an employer or not. Patients could keep or change their plan regardless of where they work. This, in turn, would increase competition and innovation in the health insurance market, resulting in better choices for everyone.

The AMA is working to reform the market by eliminating insurance company interference and regulatory/legislative meddling. These factors hamstring physicians' ability to provide care, and employers' ability to provide affordable insurance options.

The AMA plan relies on common sense and the free-market. That is how business works and what has made America the greatest economic engine in history. It's largely how life works. This is where insurance reform should begin.

Facilitating Market Innovation

Empowering people with tax credits and freedom of choice will transform today's health insurance markets. The new system will make health plans more responsive to patients and stimulate the development of new forms of insurance that better meet the wide range of needs of individuals and families. Patients desperately need more options and competition rather than fewer and fewer giant health insurance monopolies. The current system operates like the iron lung in which the patient is hopelessly encased. AMA members believe their most vulnerable patients, and nation, deserve much better.

The development of large diverse insurance pools that evenly distribute risk is imperative for the fair pricing of various plans. The federal government and Legislators understand this extremely well and have created the Federal Employees Health Benefit Plan (FEHBP)[16] to cover their own health insurance needs. The FEHBP offers the widest choice and best pricing available today. There is no reason why similar choices cannot be made available to all citizens. The key is to repeal a myriad of rules and regulations and to encourage large, actuarially sound pools to which individuals can be assigned according to their individual level of risk. This is not rocket science, but is extremely important to keep any patient from being priced out of the market, or of becoming uninsurable. Alternative means of pooling risk such as small group purchasing alliances also should be considered.

The AMA supports the development of health insurance markets that offer a wide range of coverage options that enable individuals to choose what is most appropriate and beneficial without government or industry interference. Nationwide sales and strengthened Internet-based vendors also would help to increase choice and decrease premiums. Such sales also would discourage huge variations that now occur because of individual state mandates. The AMA recognizes that for markets to function properly, it is important to establish fair ground rules; however, the huge number of state and federal health insurance market regulations has created as many problems as it has solved. Regulations intended to protect high-risk individuals typically have backfired by driving up premiums and leading a disproportionate number of young, healthy individuals to go without coverage. The AMA believes that a more rational regulatory environment would:

- Assist high-risk individuals without unduly driving up health insurance premiums for the rest of the population (ie, actuarially sound pools, plus individual assistance if needed)
- Give individuals incentives to be insured continuously to eliminate the pervasive fear of becoming uninsurable or gaming the system by only seeking coverage when sick
- Enable rather than impede private market innovations such as health savings accounts (HSAs), health reimbursement arrangements (HRAs), other forms of consumer-driven health care plans, defined contribution plans, and new forms of coverage

In particular, the AMA believes there should be greater national uniformity of market regulation across health insurance markets, regardless of type of submarket (eg, large group, small group, individual), geographic location. or type of health plan.

AMA members also believe that state variation in market regulation should be permissible as long as states demonstrate that departures from national regulations would not drive up the number of uninsured, and as long as variations do not unduly hamper the development of multistate group purchasing alliances, or create adverse selection. In short, limited state variation in market regulation should be permitted if the impact on the cost is not significant and does not make coverage unaffordable.

Risk-related subsidies such as subsidies for high-risk pools, reinsurance, and risk adjustment should be financed through general tax revenues rather than through strict community rating or premium surcharges. Strict community rating should be replaced with modified community rating, risk bands or risk corridors, and by the formation of large actuarially sound risk pools. By allowing some degree of premium variation to reflect individual factors, modified community rating strikes a balance between protecting high-risk individuals and the rest of the population.

Insured individuals also should be protected by guaranteed renewability. Allowing a fair degree of individual premium variation at the initial point of enrollment, along with guaranteed renewability, will encourage individuals to maintain their coverage. Guaranteed renewability would protect individuals from losing coverage or being singled out for premium hikes because of changes in health status.

Furthermore, insured individuals wishing to switch plans should be subject to a lesser degree of risk rating and pre-existing conditions limitations than individuals who are newly seeking coverage.

Limited reunderwriting of insured individuals who switch health plans would provide additional and powerful incentives for individuals to obtain and maintain coverage when healthy. In addition, guaranteed issue regulations should be rescinded. Guaranteed issue and community rating can backfire, especially when paired together. Attempts to lower premiums for high-risk individuals can raise premiums of low-risk individuals, reducing their enrollment and, thereby, driving up average costs and premiums. Finally, the regulatory environment should enable rather than impede private market innovation in product development and purchasing arrangements. There is such a thing as reasonable regulatory oversight, even if it rarely is seen or practiced. The AMA offers the following guide:

  Legislative and regulatory barriers to the formation and operation of group purchasing alliances in general, should be removed.
  Benefit mandates should be minimized to allow markets to determine benefit packages and permit a wide choice of coverage options.
  Any legislative and regulatory barriers to the development of multiyear insurance contracts should be identified and removed.

The AMA proposal is well-suited to incremental changes. Although the impact of revising the tax treatment of health insurance expenditures will be profound, the status quo or timid tinkering will lead only to the shifting of unconscionable cost to future generations. The AMA believes that individually owned health insurance, accomplished through fundamental changes in the current tax and individual insurance market systems, would provide the best opportunity to reverse the growth in the number of the uninsured, while increasing the health plan choices of all Americans.

The AMA proposal for health system reform fundamentally is concerned with all Americans, including those at the lowest income levels who are the most likely to be uninsured today. This plan builds upon the strengths of the current health care system and institutes reasonable reforms to correct its weaknesses. It places ownership in the hands of the individual, equalizes the tax treatment of premiums regardless of who pays, and assists those who for whatever reason are unable to pay for themselves. It contains insurance reforms that will spread risk on an actuarially sound basis, encourage competition, reduce expensive mandates, and reduce costly monopolistic behavior by insurers. Most importantly, it will begin the process of removing government and insurers from their current position between the patient and the physician.

Antitrust Reform an Important Part of Insurance Reform

The final insurance reform that is needed is to define and strictly enforce antitrust laws for insurers. The past decade has witnessed the emergence of huge for-profit health care insurance companies. These have resulted from largely unregulated mergers—more than 400 in the last 10 years. Such mergers have allowed the resultant megainsurers to increase premiums to patients, decrease reimbursement to physicians, and to record obscene levels of profit and executive pay. The American economic system depends upon an environment that spurs competition. Nothing is more anticompetitive and anti-American than a monopoly, and these huge monopolies must go.

Medical Liability Reform

The issues discussed previously represent critical pieces in the struggle to reform the United States health care system. But any true reform must include reform of a dysfunctional medical liability system that has become a national disgrace.

Every physician—from the urologist to the orthopedist, the pediatrician to the pathologist, the obstetrician to the heart surgeon—is too familiar with the specter of a medical liability lawsuit. Too often it just does not matter that physicians provide the best care humanly possible. Not all patients will be satisfied, and not all outcomes will be ideal. But that does not mean anyone made a mistake.

Unfortunately, the nation's liability system does not distinguish between poor outcomes, honest, unforeseen mistakes, and negligent practice. To be clear: If there is negligence, conscientious physicians are the first to demand that the patient should receive fair compensation. If there is no negligence (and here the author talking about knowing the difference between a bad outcome and a negligent one), then the physician should not be subject to a lawsuit that not only will cost tens of thousands of dollars to defend, but costs the physician priceless time away from his or her practice, patients, and family. The nation also would save as much as $126 billion if liability reforms, including a $250,000 cap on noneconomic damages, were in place nationally. Everywhere that tort reforms, including caps on noneconomic damages have been enacted, improved access has followed.

WHAT WOULD THE AMERICAN MEDICAL ASSOCIATION LIKE YOU TO DO?

Physicians, patients, and community leaders have said that ensuring the availability of health care for Americans is the number one domestic issue facing this country. It is no secret that there are 47 million uninsured Americans, and that those who do have coverage live in constant fear of losing that insurance. AMA members are pleased many of the presidential candidates are beginning to address the issue. Their help is needed,, but the physicians and patients of America must lead this change. A patient must choose and own his of her own insurance policy and be able to see the physician of his or her choice. This means patients must help design the health care system of the future and not accept whatever some political advisors think will bring their candidate a majority of votes. One's health and the health of loved ones are the most important issues. One must not allow it to be decided by television sound bites, unrealistic political promises that ignore the wisdom of experience.

At the risk of being too persistent, the author wishes to re-emphasize the fact that the AMA's birth more than 150 years ago was the professional response of physicians to a national need to improve the quality of medical care. Today, the AMA is calling for another outburst of national attention and national action to make certain that access to quality care remains a top priority for candidates and the American public. When this happens, candidates hopefully will have no choice but to confront it with concrete ideas and practical solutions.

AMA members want to enlist physician and patient help in making sure the candidates remember that when it comes to health care, a serious plan of action is needed, not a news conference dog and pony show. The AMA is engaged in a campaign to ensure that the candidates are intercepted in the key primary states, in Washington, DC, and at all points in between. AMA members are talking to community leaders who have the influence and know-how. They are reaching out in periodicals such as this to reach the best clinical minds in the country so all patients can be reached.

There is a choice. The nation can indulge in another round of platitudes and procrastination, or it can confront the issue of serious health care system reform. Reform that extricates government and insurers from their current position between the patient and the physician and returns insurance ownership to the patient and decision making to the patient in concert with the physician. Let the candidates this year and next year know where physicians stand. Bring the AMA's message to neighbors, friends, pastors, and school superintendents.

Be an activist. Begin at home. Those who have sons or daughters between the ages of 19 and 24 should make sure they understand what is at stake, and that they get adequate coverage.

Together, this problem can be solved. Together, a better America can be built.

The author is nearing the end of his AMA tenure as immediate past president, but his voice is as strong as ever for patients and the medical profession. Together, the trust and confidence patients have given physicians can be used for the betterment of this great nation.

REFERENCES

1. FDR and polio—Campobello. Franklin and Eleanor Roosevelt Institute. Available at: http://www.feri.org/arcfaVes/polio/default.cfm. Accessed December 20, 2007.
2. Iron lung. University of Virginia. Available at: http://liistorical.hsl.virginia.edu/ironlung/pg4.cfm. Accessed December 20, 2007.
3. The TIME 100: Jonas Salk. Available at: http://www.time.com/time/timeIOO/scientist/profile/salk.html. Accessed December 20, 2007.
4. AMA launches multi-million dollar campaign to cover the uninsured [press release]. American Medical Association; August 23, 2007.
5. Income climbs, poverty stabilizes, uninsured rate increases [press release]. US Census Bureau; August 9, 2007.
6. A survey conducted for the AMA by Harris Interactive in found that 85 percent of Americans trust their physician—a figure far higher than any other profession. On file with author. August 2007.
7. See Supra note 5.
8. Fact sheet 5. Uninsurance facts and figures: the uninsured are sicker and die sooner. The Institute of Medicine. Available at: http://www.iom.edu/CMS/17645.aspx. Accessed December 20, 2007.
9. The uninsured and their access to health care. Kaiser Family Foundation fact sheet. Available at: http://www.kff.org/iumisiiredfapload/The-Uninsured-and-Their-Access-to-Health-Care-Oct-2004.pdf.
10. Institute of Medicine. Hidden costs. Values lost: uninsurance in America. The National Academies Press; 2003.
11. See 2007. Kaiser Family Foundation employer health benefits report. Available at: http://www.kff.org/msurance/7672/.
12. History of health insurance benefits. Employee benefits research institute fact sheet. Available at: http://wttrw.ebri.org/publications/facts/index.cfm?fa=0302fact.

13. Internal Revenue Service. Tax guide to fringe bene-fits. Publication 15-B (for 2007). Available at: http://www.irs.gov/pub/irs-pdf/p15b.pdf.

14. Expanding health insurance: the AMA proposal for reform. Available at: http://www.ama-assn.org/amal/pub/upload/mm/363/ehil012.pdf.

15. E.g. attempts in Illinois and California are two of the most recent attempts for a state to engage in wide-spread policymaking without having the funding mechanisms to pay for the policies.

16. US Office of Personnel Management Web site. Available at: http://www.opm.gov/insure/liealtlVabout/index.asp.

Residency Training: Where Do We Go from Here

Robert R. Bahnson, MD, FACS

KEYWORDS

• Urology • Education • Curriculum • Residency

Residency training in urologic surgery should change to an educational experience driven by outcomes instead of process. The needs analysis for curriculum modification has been completed and defines the competencies (enduring skills) of the complete physician. The challenge now rests with organizational leaders of urology to design programs that ensure the acquisition of these characteristics and conserve time and economic resources.

Curriculum change in urologic residency training programs should occur because health care in America has changed. Specialization of physicians, acceleration in total spending, and an insatiable demand for service requires adjustments in a society with finite resources. Doctors have traditionally designed curricula for postgraduate residency training with minimal attention to the ramifications of length of training and its associated costs. Because we recognize the substantial shortage in the urologic workforce, our plans for modification of training should improve access to urologic service delivery while preserving our precious resources of time and money. The subsequent opinions in this article are those of the author. The recommendations have prejudice and assume the reader agrees that demand and expenditure for urologic service are going to increase over the next 3 decades. No effort, other than references, is made to document or substantiate these assumptions.

CURRENT STATUS OF RESIDENCY TRAINING

At present, the potential number of board-certified urologists is limited by the number of available positions in Accreditation Council for Graduate Medical Education (ACGME)–accredited residency training programs in urology. The Residency Review Committee (RRC) for urology is not limited in the number of training programs it may approve. The RRC only judges the quality of the program and its ability to train residents who are competent to practice the specialty of urology independently. Theoretically, and in practice, urologic services can be provided by practitioners who are neither board-certified nor a graduate of an accredited training program. How is this possible? As long as the state medical boards are willing to provide medical licenses and hospitals are given the authority of credentialing their staff members, the desperate need for urologic practitioners is likely to lead hospitals to structure their bylaws to permit individuals without board certification or a certificate from an accredited training program to practice urology. It is this author's opinion that in an information age that promotes consumerism, the demand for physicians with board certification and documentation of maintenance of certification (MOC) is only going to increase and exacerbate the shortage of urologic specialty care. A second, equally powerful, driving force behind the current diminished urologic service availability is money. The reimbursement of professional service has undergone steady erosion since the last quarter of the twentieth century, and the diminution in value of surgical fees has been striking.[1] The response has not been surprising as surgeons (not just urologic) abandon the hospitals and their operating rooms for ambulatory surgery centers (ASCs) or office-based practices and procedures. This change in *modus operandi*

Department of Urology, Ohio State University, 456 West 10th Avenue, Columbus, OH 43210, USA
E-mail address: robert.bahnson@osumc.edu

Urol Clin N Am 36 (2009) 73–77
doi:10.1016/j.ucl.2008.08.009

provides the additional gratuitous benefit of increasing throughput, improving case mix, capturing facility fees, and limiting emergency room call and medical malpractice liability. Proof of this principle is confirmed in the case logs of urologists who are recertifying at 10- and 20-year intervals after the first attainment of board certification.[2] The experiences reported by these practitioners are heavily weighted toward low-acuity cases that can be performed rapidly and with minimal risk.

THE CASE FOR A CHANGE IN RESIDENCY TRAINING

The American Urologic Association (AUA) Board of Directors appointed a task force in October of 2005 to assess the current status of residency training and to explore the potential for modification of training. The constituencies represented in these meetings included the AUA, the American Board of Urology (ABU), the RRC for urology, private practice urologists, and residency program directors. What follows is a recapitulation of the white paper authored by John McConnell and published first in the AUA news.[3]

The objectives of the strategic planning group were to (1) define the strengths and weaknesses of urology graduate medical education at this time; (2) define the potential threats to the current training model, including subspecialization, and external competitive threats involving other branches of medicine; (3) define the likely future state of urologic practice; (4) define the urologic training required to prepare urologists for the future state of urologic practice; (5) make specific recommendations to the AUA Board of Directors, the ABU, the Urology Residency Committee, the Society of University Urologists, the Society of University Chairs and Program Directors, and AUA subspecialty societies to close the gap between the current and future state of training and; (6) develop strategies to communicate the planning group's recommendations to all stakeholders.

The need for change in residency training has been illustrated by recertification operative logs submitted to the ABU. These data indicate that the average urologist at the time of certification and at the time of recertification performs a relatively low number of major urologic operations. A urologist who performs one radical prostatectomy per year or 0.5 radical cystectomy per year is in the top percentile of case volume. Office-based procedures now constitute more than one half of total urologic procedures (eg, cystoscopies, prostate biopsies). This discrepancy between the reported surgical logs of practitioners and the surgical case logs of residents in training promoted a healthy discussion as to whether the current residency program structure prepared urologists well for what they would actually be doing in practice. As we assess the needs of the population for urologic services, it is clear that changes in training should be considered to address future need for urologic service. The current state of urologic practice is a changing landscape. Thirty-five years ago, solo practitioners and small groups of urologists predominated in the marketplace. Perceived economic advantage has led to consolidation in larger markets, and these megagroups often recruit fellowship-trained urologists who cover subspecialty areas. Even in these large groups, however, the leaders of practices desire broad training for their urologist members because they are often required to cover common urologic emergencies and care issues for the group when on call. This increased specialization has seen a parallel increasing role for midlevel providers, such as physician's assistants and nurse practitioners. Although these midlevel practitioners may provide an opportunity for a urologist to focus on a surgical practice, others view them as a potential threat to the specialty. In addition, urogyncology, radiation oncology, medical oncology, interventional radiology, and reproductive endocrinology compete with urology in many markets across numerous disease states. The panel agreed that although a fellowship-trained urologic specialist may be the ideal way to meet the competitive threat successfully, it is impractical to think that urology can train sufficient subspecialists to meet the volume demands. The broadly trained urologist in most practice settings must be able to provide adequate urologic care to a wide range of patients and disease processes, with the probable exception of major pediatric urologic surgery cases.

Urology has typically attracted the best and the brightest medical students to the specialty. We generally fill all available urology positions in residency programs, and the specialty continues to be attractive because of the mix between surgical and medical management approaches. The planning group, however, concluded that surgery is the key element in attractiveness of the specialty. It was thought that a two-tiered training approach would make urology a much less attractive specialty to medical students if there was a suggestion that some would perform far fewer surgical procedures. The planning group took note that many medical school graduates face educational debts of more than $100,000, and $150,000 in some cases, when they begin residency training. They pragmatically recognized that a 5- to 6-year training program may pose a barrier to students when they compare urology with fields that only require 3 years of training. The planning group expressed a strong desire to keep urology more attractive by potentially limiting the length of training and to promote diversity in the specialty by appealing to and recruiting women and underrepresented minorities.

The planning group also reviewed the issue of certificates of added qualification (CAQs), and they did not reach a consensus. The ABU continues to review and consider CAQs based on their merit. Although the planning group did not reach a consensus, they did unanimously support the importance of fellowship training to the future of urology. They recognized that fellowships enhanced the overall quality of a training program and aided in faculty recruitment and retention. The future of academic urology depends on the fellowship pipeline. Acknowledging the value and importance of fellowship training led the group to consider the possibility of shortening the overall time requirement to achieve specialization. It was thought that urology could develop a clearly defined core curriculum and advance those interested in specialization and differentiation toward that area before completion of residency. The RRC and program directors have articulated a clear willingness to consider a flexible curriculum that would give advanced placement credit for a portion of fellowship training to those individuals who focused their penultimate and ultimate years of training on that particular discipline.

In an effort to assist core curriculum planning and revision, the RRC leadership has re-evaluated the residency program's index cases percentile requirements. After grouping certain types of cases into several categories, the RRC has suggested minimums of surgical experience for accreditation. This effort has already undergone several discussions, and a presentation for clarification of these changes was made at the June 2007 meeting of the RRC. The planning group also thought that there was an opportunity for better coordination of the early residency experience. Defining more precisely the requirements and expectations of the preliminary urology experience may create an opportunity for more elective time in later years. The panel concluded with a series of specific recommendations:

1. Communicate that a two-tiered model in the United States is not in the best interest of patients or the specialty.
2. Develop a national core curriculum to include cognitive and manipulative skills.
3. Begin to define the knowledge and skills that should be acquired during core versus fellowship training.
4. Put urology program directors in charge of the first postgraduate year.
5. Make the last 2 years of residency flexible after core competencies are developed.
6. Move away from all residents needing equal surgical logs.
7. Integrate the chief residency year into fellowship training for those who wish to pursue subspecialization.
8. Develop a fellowship program directors' organization.
9. Define who controls the quality of the fellowships.
10. Reinforce the importance of the research experience.
11. Develop electives for residents headed for academic careers to develop skills in teaching, research, writing, and grantsmanship.
12. Put ongoing assessment of urologic training into a continuous quality improvement model and repeat national assessments periodically.

TOWARD A NEW PROGRAM FOR REQUIREMENTS FOR RESIDENCY TRAINING IN UROLOGY

It is appropriate and timely to design a new curriculum for training specialists in urologic surgery. Current programs have gaps and variability that limit the educational experience of the residents. The change should follow the recommendations of educators who have shown the value of backward design. Steven R. Covey, in the *Seven Habits of Highly Effective People*, emphasizes the rationale behind a backward curriculum design. "To begin with the end in mind means to start with a clear understanding of your destination. It means to know where you are going so that you better understand where you are now so that the steps you take are always in the right direction."[4] Why is this termed *backward design*? This design emphasizes that the stages are logical but that they go against our natural habits. Educators often jump to content in learning strategy ideas before clarifying performance objectives for students. By thinking through the assessments up front, we ensure greater alignment of our objectives and means. The stages in the backward design of a curriculum are as follows. First, we identify the desired results. In a sense, this has been done for us by the ACGME Outcomes Project, in which the definition of a successful physician is rooted in the acquisition of core competencies. The second step in backward design is to determine the acceptable evidence that is available for the acquisition of the desired results. Once this has been determined, educators can then plan learning experiences and instruction. Specifically, a curriculum design should define what residents know, understand, and are able to do. As the curriculum design proceeds, knowledge of Bloom's taxonomy must be taken into consideration. In 1996, Benjamin Bloom headed a group of educational psychologists who developed a classification of levels of intellectual behavior important in learning. This became a taxonomy, including three overlapping domains: the cognitive, psychomotor, and affective. Categories within the cognitive domain include knowledge, comprehension, application, analysis, and synthesis. Bloom's taxonomy emphasizes that the learners have different approaches and backgrounds that they bring to the learning situation. Educators must recognize that students are different. They think differently because of differences in their cognitive domain. Their values and their feelings are different, and this is a reflection of their affective domain. They act and respond differently to instructions because of differences that they all possess in their behavioral domains.

The needs analysis has defined the core competencies that are the knowledge, skills, and attributes required of the successful urology resident. The learners are the residents, and educators must take into consideration different learning styles in the cognitive, affective, and behavioral domains to help foster the acquisition of these competencies.

The ACGME general competencies include patient care, medical knowledge, practice-based learning and improvement, interpersonal and communication skills, professionalism, and systems-based practice. As we establish the curriculum priorities for acquisition of these competencies, we must define those core skills that are enduring and are required of every resident. In addition, it is important to identify those skills that are important to know and periodically do and, finally, consider those skills and knowledge that are worth being familiar with. The final stage in curriculum design is the planning of learning experiences and instructions. This requires a recitation of which learning activities are going to equip residents with the needed knowledge and skills. Examples of such activities include lectures and didactic presentations, small group discussions and seminars, demonstrations, and resident interviews with objective standardized clinical evaluations (OSCEs). Films that include instructional materials and require student interaction and problem-based learning modules similar to those that have been incorporated into medical school curricula are

needed. Finally, the ACGME has considered the idea of portfolios, in which residents throughout training keep journals that are written reflections of their interaction and learning experiences. Educators know the resources best suited to accomplish these learning goals. They include trained faculty, standards of practice, modules in the core competencies, interactive software, standardized patients, and coaching and feedback. For the overall design to be coherent and effective, it must take advantage of skill building. This is best performed from low-risk tasks, to intermediate-risk tasks, to, ultimately, high-risk tasks. This promotes increased skills building as residents go from simple to complex procedures, increasing their sophistication of application. The learning experiences must be engaging and diverse and must create depth and breadth of understanding of the specialty of urology.

THE NEW PRODUCT

The best physicians are problem solvers. They integrate medical knowledge, experience, and familiarity with ancillary services to improve the lives of the patients they care for. These practitioners unfailingly put patient's interests ahead of their own and subscribe to truth telling in a manner that is culturally tolerant and individually sensitive.

The efforts of many have defined the core competencies of the physician, and they codify the desired result of a training program. We have a proved effective method for assessing the trainees' acquisition of urologic knowledge. The in-training examination, qualifying examination, and certifying examination administered by the ABU provide a validated measure of this core competency. Measurement of professionalism, interpersonal and communication skills, practice-based learning and improvement, and systems-based practice requires further effort.

Most all residency programs are geographically juxtaposed to centers of higher learning. We need to access our expert colleagues in education to help us develop the assessment and instructional tools for propagation and inculcation of these core competencies. Perhaps the most important of all changes is the reduction in total training time for individuals who pursue fellowship training. This challenges us as educators to define a urologic core curriculum with broad exposure to the specialized domains of urology. The American College of Surgeons (ACS) has worked diligently to develop the fundamentals of surgery residents' curriculum. This would be applicable to all medical school graduates who pursue surgical training. Interestingly, this paradigm would assume that those individuals would acquire cognitive skills in their final year of medical school, including principles of perioperative care, wound healing, fluid and electrolytes, surgical infections, surgical emergency, nutrition, basic skills training, and professional competencies (eg, communication, systems-based practice, practice-based learning).

The fundamentals of the surgery curriculum in the first postgraduate year would include the following modules: advanced principles of perioperative care, disorders of wound healing, blood products, fluids and electrolytes, pain management, surgical management of emergencies, anesthesiology, surgical infections and antibiotics, nutrition, sepsis, trauma and resuscitation, renal and hepatic failure, cardiac and pulmonary emergencies, principles of surgical oncology, palliative care, informed consent, ethics, principles of evidence-based practice, outcomes assessment, professionalism, interpersonal communication, practice-based learning, and systems-based practice. The core training program would also include a skill acquisition model using simulation. This would begin with knowledge acquisition through self-study, which would be the cognitive phase. It would progress to a fixation phase using simulators and subsequent supervised performance with live patients. The final assessment of the acquisition of the skill would be the autonomous phase with independent performance.

The core urology program (postgraduate years 2–3) would then build on the surgical platform to advance the resident to a level of competency in general urology. The final phase of training (postgraduate years 4–5) could vary depending on the career goals of the individual trainee. Those wishing to enter practice would complete training with a focus on increasing independence in practice experience and teaching with electives in areas of interest. Urology residents with interest in a specific domain of urology could elect to spend more focused effort on rotations in that field and enter fellowship ready for their highly advanced training modules in that discipline.

THE OUTCOME

A shift in urologic surgical education is not going to occur with rapidity. The evolution is going to be deliberate and is going to encounter obstacles known and unknown. We can be enthusiastic, however, and embrace these changes because our specialty has been characterized by physician leaders with the power to change lives. Urologists willingly have and continue to pledge themselves to the privilege and necessity of training those who are going to replace them.

REFERENCES

1. DeGroote R. The economics of managed care reimbursement: a rationale for nonparticipation. Bull Am Coll Surg 2007;92(4):28–36.
2. Carroll PR, Albertson PC, Smith JA, et al. Volume of major surgeries performed by recent and more senior graduates from North American urology training programs. J Urol 2006;175(4):1.
3. McConnell JD, Clayman RV, Flanigan RC, et al. The future of urology and urologic education in America. AUA News 2007.
4. Covey S. The 7 Habits of Highly Effective People. Free Press; 1990.

Certification, Recertification, and Maintenance: Continuing to Learn

Linda M. Dairiki Shortliffe, MD[a,b,c,*]

KEYWORDS
- Certification • Recertification • American Board of Urology
- Medical specialties

THE UPWARD SPIRAL

Renewal is the principle—and the process—that empowers us to move on an upward spiral of growth and change, of continuous improvement. ...[As] we grow and develop on this upward spiral, we must show diligence in the process of renewal by educating and obeying our conscience. An increasingly educated conscience will propel us along the path of personal freedom, security, wisdom, and power. Moving along the upward spiral ...to keep progressing...we must learn, commit, and do...and learn, commit, and do again.[1]

When Steven Covey published "The 7 Habits of Highly Effective People" in 1989, he was not speaking to the medical community but was addressing people as a management guru on personal development. Since that time, we have had our own medical spiral and some may believe it has been down rather than up. The rapidity of changes over the past two decades is enormous. Although many medical practitioners feel that regulation and compliance issues are directed only at the medical profession as a part of this, this is not the case. The medical community is one of many areas in which regulation has occurred.

The United States is a leader in medicine, but this was not always the case, and some may argue that it is not the case of the present or future. The pre-eminent position of American medicine is related to the regulation of medical education and specialization that occurred in the early part of the twentieth century. It was not until the 1920s that "American medical education had evolved from the worst in industrialized civilization to the very best...the marvel of the industrial world."[2] In the early 1900s, US medical schools had few standards, and education in scientific practice and knowledge lagged behind European counterparts, especially Germany and France. Many medical schools were being run primarily for profit. Abraham Flexner pointed out these deficiencies in a report in 1910 entitled "Medical Education in the United States and Canada" ("the Flexner Report") commissioned by the Carnegie Foundation for the Advancement of Teaching. Although such reports are usually dry reading, the Flexner Report instigated revolutionary change in medical education. This revolution resulted in standardization of medical school curricula.

Around this time, medical specialties also emerged, among which was urology. David Innes Williams, a renowned urologic surgeon at St. Peter's Hospital and the Hospital for Sick Children at Great Ormond Street, has defined a specialty. "A speciality [sic] has both a technical and a social dimension. Technically, it is defined by an acknowledged territory, a corpus of relevant

a Department of Urology, Stanford University School of Medicine, CA, USA
b Department of Urology, S-287, Stanford University Medical Center MC: 5118, 300 Pasteur Drive, Stanford, CA 94305-5118, USA
c Lucile Salter Packard Children's Hospital, Stanford, CA, USA
* Department of Urology, S-287, Stanford University Medical Center MC: 5118, 300 Pasteur Drive, Stanford, CA 94305-5118.
E-mail address: lindashortliffe@stanford.edu

Urol Clin N Am 36 (2009) 79–83
doi:10.1016/j.ucl.2008.08.001

knowledge, and a range of skills not readily acquired by the profession at large. The emergence of a surgical specialty was most often triggered by the skills required after the invention of a new instrument or a new operative procedure. Socially, a specialty can be seen to exist when there is a body of practitioners who devote the greater part of their time to a limited field who are recognized by designated appointments as providing a special service and who organize specialist societies and journals."[3]

Although urology branched from general surgery in the United States and most of Europe, in Great Britain urology remained a subspecialty of general surgery. Before the turn of the century, urology was recognized as a specialty separate from general surgery in the United States and most of Europe. This interesting history of disparate urologic development is attributed to the differing administrative structure with a national health system dominated by consultants of the two Royal Colleges, strength of the General Practice sector, and lack of a supportive university system.[3]

After the restructure and regulation of medical schools that occurred in response to the Flexner Report, medical specialty boards started to appear. The stated purpose of these Boards was to improve standards of training and protect the public from "superficial training and commercialism."[2] Before their appearance, postgraduate medical education (residencies) lacked uniformity of content, had varying supervision, and varied in duration from weeks to months to years. The American Board of Ophthalmology was established in 1917, followed by the American Board of Otolaryngology in 1924, the Board of Obstetrics and Gynecology in 1930, the Board of Urology in 1935 (along with Orthopaedic Surgery, Pediatrics, and Radiology the same year), and the American Board of Surgery in 1937. Currently, 24 incorporated Boards exist, all of which are members of the American Board of Medical Specialties (ABMS), and one or more of the current boards certifies almost 90% of practicing physicians.

The Liaison Committee for Graduate Medical was established in 1972 as a private regulatory body for graduate medical education. It was succeeded by the Accreditation Council of Graduate Medical Education, which was established by consensus of the academic medical community as an independent accrediting organization in 1981 for postgraduate residency programs in the United States. Although medical school and postgraduate residency growth was originally disorganized and somewhat chaotic, public notice produced private regulation.

As a specialty, urology continues to evolve, with its practitioners integrating medical, surgical, technologic, imaging, and pharmacologic discoveries into new means for diagnosis, management, treatment, and prevention of genitourinary problems. The core of urologic diagnostics, management, and treatment always has involved medical and surgical components, but these areas and components of imaging, pharmacology, chemotherapy, and endoscopy have advanced in complexity and scope. Urologic imaging is no longer limited to retrograde pyelography, intravenous urography, and voiding cystourethrograms but encompasses ultrasonography, nuclear renography, CT, MRI, positron emission tomography, and molecular imaging, with decision analysis for selecting the optimal studies for the occasion. Treatment of advanced prostate cancer is no longer limited to diethylstilbestrol and radiation but includes new surgical and chemotherapeutic options, hormonal manipulation, radiation, and cyberknife. Pharmacologic choices for infection, impotence, prostatic enlargement, and incontinence are numerous.

Further subspecialization continues. With the explosive advances in medical knowledge and technology, specialists in areas previously unrecognized, such as trauma, critical care, endovascular surgical neuroradiology, and molecular genetics pathology, are common and sometimes required for hospitals. The landscape that composes the corpus for urology is reflected in the recent American Board of Urology (ABU) listing of the scope of urology, which includes but is not limited to the following: cognitive areas, such as ethics and professionalism, evidence-based medicine, perioperative care, wound healing/management, adrenal disease, benign renal disease, endocrinology, calculus disease, benign prostate disease, infertility female pelvic medicine and surgery, geriatric urology, infectious disease, neurourology and voiding dysfunction, urethral and ureteral obstructions, oncology, pediatric urology, renovascular disease, sexual dysfunction (male/female), renal transplantation, trauma, basic genitourinary pathology, and relevant diagnostic and technical skills, such as imaging (physics, diagnostic and therapeutic), open surgical skills/techniques, endourology, shock wave lithotripsy, laparoscopy, and urodynamics.[4]

Urologic specialty societies, such as pediatrics, oncology, endourology, sexual medicine, female and neurourology, basic science, genitourinary reconstructions, and transplantation and renal surgery, also reflect the expanded areas of practice and interest. This superspecialization trend represents further differentiation within urology. This is a normal response to growth of a body of knowledge that is subdivided into multiple areas of specialties. In Williams' terms, each of these areas represents the embodiment of speciality with technical and social dimensions. The trend is apparent in the United States and Europe.[5,6]

It is not surprising that more extensive regulation of the practitioner after certification has emerged to protect the public. In 1986, legislation created the National Practitioner Data Bank; in 1996, the Secretary of the US Department of Health and Human Services—acting through the Office of Inspector General—created the Healthcare Integrity and Protection Data Bank as directed by the Health Insurance Portability and Accountability Act to combat fraud and abuse in health insurance and health care delivery. Both acts were instigated by practitioners crossing state lines to avoid discovery, and some of the current interest in recertification and maintenance of certification requirements is probably the result of the emphasis on medical error recognition. The stated purpose for creating the National Practitioner Data Bank was the "increasing occurrence of medical malpractice litigation and the need to improve the quality of medical care had become nationwide problems that warranted greater efforts than any individual State could undertake. The intent was to improve the quality of health care by encouraging state licensing boards, hospitals and other health care entities, and professional societies to identify and discipline those who engage in unprofessional behavior; and to restrict the ability of incompetent physicians...to move from State to State without disclosure or discovery of previous medical malpractice payment and adverse action history."[7] Perhaps this is an example of rules being made after predecessors break a trust.

Others with less onerous responsibilities have a similar history of regulation. As a result of concerns not unlike those discussed, the regulation of truck drivers and airline pilots occurred with expansion of services and formation of the US Department of Transportation. In 1934, Lubin, a member of President Roosevelt's Advisory Committee on Federal Coordination of Railroads, became interested in motor vehicles and trucking and warned that 8 hours or more of driving created hazardous driving circumstances. When addressing the American Trucking Association, ne noted that lack of self-regulation would lead to federal regulation.[8] A 1982 study estimated that driver error was the major cause of truck accidents 80% of the time.[8] Not until 1992 did truck drivers have to pass written and driving tests to meet minimum federal standards, and prior training ranged from 150 to 610 hours without standardized licensing. These changes were instigated by the fact that large truck drivers needed only a routine driver's license in 18 states, and they could easily obtain licenses in multiple states and avoid suspensions by spreading violations among the different licenses.

Long before concerns for regulating or mandating educational updating were entertained, individuals interested in continuing medical education focused on why and how physicians continue to learn after completion of their formal training and the need for lifelong learning.[9,10] In personal essays on those remarkable stars of medical practice, discovery, and innovation, Manning and DeBakey found that these individuals have a "passion" for learning. Dr. A. McGehee Harvey, former chairman of the department of medicine at The Johns Hopkins University School of Medicine and physician-in-chief of The Johns Hopkins Hospital, stated "To be a good physician...[It] is a matter of developing the habit of learning so that it becomes second nature an not something you turn on and off at certain times...Education must be pursued actively, not through the passive receipt of information distilled by someone else...A teacher can provide motivation and an environment for learning, but it is still up to the student to be an active learner."[10]

Dr. Michael DeBakey, internationally renowned cardiac surgeon, director of the DeBakey Heart Center, previous chairman of the department of surgery, chancellor of the Baylor School of Medicine, and chairman of President Johnson's Commission on Heart Disease, Cancer, and Stroke, recalled an incident from his childhood. "When I was a very young boy, my Father took me on a hunting trip, and when he set me down in the field, he said, 'Now stay right here; I won't be far away.' He would go a short distance...returning every little while to bring back the ducks that he had shot. On one such occasion...I had my hands behind my back, and he said, 'What's wrong with your hands?'...I had to reveal my hands, which were bloody. He was immediately alarmed and asked, 'What did you do? Did you cut yourself?' I confessed that I had taken a knife out ...and had opened the ducks...'I wanted to find out how they fly,' I explained. Shortly after, my Father read me a book about birds flying." This episode emphasizes, however, that passion and active learning must reside in the learner, and support of a teacher is needed for the best learning.

Perhaps what does not reside in the learner is just as important. Research has documented that students who fail often lack self-reflection. Although there may be indicators of lacking knowledge or poor performance, these students may be unlikely to foresee it, although others may.[11] Active and proscribed educational activities may need to be required for these individuals to acquire new knowledge or learn to perform at improved levels. Research on the adoption and diffusion of innovations and new knowledge shows that personal and environmental characteristics are important to this process. Individuals have varying degrees of resistance to change or adopting new ideas that may or may not be scientifically based. With adoption of any new idea or innovation, predictable categories of group behavior have been studied, and patterns of adoption fall into categories: innovators, early adopters, early majority, late majority, and laggards.[12] Each of these categories has its own personality and behavioral characteristics, which is an issue that may create haphazard adoption of new practices.

Although past practitioners' education after residency was from formal educational courses, organized educational meetings and conferences, and literature, current education has many additional formats, such as multimedia that include telephone, radio, television, cable, and Internet. These formats have increased our capabilities for improving knowledge and communication and have created a "flat world."[13] All of this potential education is based on self-motivation and personal willingness to learn and adopt new knowledge. Two trends, the first being the ability to track quality and results through information technology and second being the recognition that individual error and failure may be prevented, have created a need for improved surveillance of physician continuing medical education.

Although the ABU did not invent or ask for "maintenance of certification," the concept maintains the original mission of the specialty Boards. Maintenance of certification is a concept that was created by the ABMS in 1999 in response to increasing public scrutiny and awareness that physicians keep up with medical advances. The concept encompasses recertification and several elements that document a practitioner's continuing involvement in medical education. The ABMS is asking physicians to fulfill four components: evidence of professional standing, evidence of commitment to lifelong learning and involvement in periodic self-assessment processes, evidence of cognitive expertise, and evidence of evaluation and performance in practice. The ABU is judging professional standing by peer review and judging evidence of cognitive expertise with certification or recertification testing. Findings will be used as evidence of commitment to periodic self-assessment. As a result, the first two of these

components—evidence of professional standing and cognitive expertise—are already accomplished in the initial ABU certification and recertification process. The latter two areas of regular periodic self-assessment processes and evidence of evaluation and performance in practice are the areas in which the ABMS is requesting more documentation. The ABU will be using practice assessment protocols based on current urologic clinical guidelines to perform evaluation of performance in practice. Diplomates will perform self-review of a series of their personal cases in a specific area and compare their practice to those managed according to accepted guidelines. Beginning in 2007, physicians with time-limited certificates will enter the maintenance of certification process in the year in which they recertify (**Table 1**).

The consequence of lack of compliance after original agreement with ABMS plans would be forfeiture of ABMS membership. As the public increasingly looks for quality measures on which to evaluate physicians, being board certified is one of the measures of quality that we hope to establish and continue. Ultimately, the ABMS is concerned about patient care, and its role is to protect patients and improve standards of physician training. At the time that maintenance of certification is implemented, approximately 80% of practicing urologists will be involved in the program. Maintenance of certification gives a false impression of the process, because "maintenance" fails to construe the process leading to active acquisition of new knowledge and skill since original certification, which is the important part of this process. As members of the ABMS, the Trustees of the ABU will develop a process that allows diplomats to demonstrate their ongoing efforts to advance their expertise in urology as the specialty evolves. As new urologic or urology-pertinent practice guidelines and recommendations are generated, practice assessment protocols will allow practitioners to demonstrate their knowledge in areas that they select. This assessment will affirm that board-certified urologists are professionals who hold the welfare and benefit of their patients in esteem.

The history of the development of urology and its certification in the United States is part of the development of surgical differentiation and subspecialization. The original drivers for medical certification were concern for quality of patient care and public protection by requiring individuals to demonstrate appropriate and specific training and accomplishment in their area of practice. The drivers for recertification and maintenance of certification are an ever-changing and expanding knowledge base, public awareness of medical

Table 1
Maintenance of certification requirements

Requirements	Level 1 (Year 2)	Level 2 (Year 4)	Level 3 (Year 6)	Level 4 (Years 7–9)
Complete application online	Yes	Update demographic information	Update demographic information	Update demographic information
ABU office verify licensure	Yes	Yes	Yes	Yes
ABU office complete peer review	No	Yes	No	Yes
Candidate: complete online practice assessment protocol	Yes	Yes	Yes	Yes
Candidate: submit documentation of 90 hours of continuing medical education	No	Yes	No	Yes
Candidate: submit 6-month electronic practice log	No	No	No	Yes
Candidate: computer-based closed-book examination	No	No	No	Yes

Data from Stuart S. Howards, MD, Executive Secretary of the American Board of Urology, written communication, 2008.

error, and medical commercialism in a world in which the public has the potential for knowledge equal to or greater than that of the practitioner. Dissemination of new medical practice and knowledge cannot be based on random likelihood of whether a physician does or does not acquire knowledge for reasons of passion, personality characteristics, or self-reflection. The baseline must be higher.

REFERENCES

1. Covey SR. The 7 habits of highly effective people. New York: Simon & Schuster; 1989.
2. Ludmerer KM. Time to heal: American medical education from the turn of the century to the era of managed care. New York: Oxford University Press; 1999.
3. Innes Williams D. The development of urology as a speciality in Britain. BJU Int 1999;84(6):587–94.
4. American Board of Urology. The certification process; (annual brochure), 2007.
5. Debruyne FMJ. Subspecialty certification in urology: a European perspective. Nat Clin Pract Urol 2006; 3(12):625.
6. Flanigan RC. Subspecialty certification in urology: a US perspective. Nat Clin Pract Urol 2006;3(10):509.
7. National Practitioner Data Bank.
8. Whitnah DR. US Department of transportation: a reference history. Westport (CT): Greenwood Press; 1998. p. 228.
9. Manning P, DeBakey L. Medicine: preserving the passion. New York: Springer-Verlag; 1987.
10. Manning P, DeBakey L. Medicine: preserving the passion in the 21st century. 2nd edition. New York: Springer-Verlag; 2004.
11. Cleland J, Arnold R, Chesser A. Failing finals is often a surprise for the student but not the teacher: identifying difficulties and supporting students with academic difficulties. Med Teach 2005;27(6):504–8.
12. Rogers E. Diffusion of innovations. New York: Free Press; 2003.
13. Friedman T. The world is flat: a brief history of the twenty-first century. New York: Farrar, Straus and Giroux; 2005.

The Sad and Bleak Future for Urology Funding at the National Institutes of Health

Lars M. Ellison, MD[a],*, Carl A. Olsson, MD[b]

KEYWORDS
- Funding • Research • Urology

The bulk of federal funding for medical research is delivered through the National Institutes of Health (NIH). Other players in the field include, but are not limited to Department of Defense (DOD), the Department of Veterans Affairs (VA), the Centers for Disease Control and Prevention (CDC), the Department of Energy (DOE), and the National Science Foundation (NSF). Of the $30 billion for medical research in the 2007 budget, $28 billion were allocated to NIH.[1] It is quite clear, therefore, that the lifeblood of medical researchers is intimately tied to the vitality of NIH.

Federal funding of medical research is coordinated through the annual discretionary budget review process. Unlike direct spending programs (entitlements such as Medicare, Medicaid, and Social Security) that have legal mandate to collect and spend funds, the annual discretionary spending review process requires prior approval by subcommittees and committees of the House and Senate, subject to final approval of the president.[2] The net result of this process is that the budget for NIH varies from year to year. Overall, despite the organic nature of an appropriated budget, NIH has enjoyed annual growth throughout its entire history up until 2004.[3,4]

When examined from the viewpoint of many years or decades, one would anticipate the budget is likely to continue its upward growth trajectory. Therefore, from this long-range perspective, the president and the legislature would rightly anticipate a robust future for the global leadership role the United States has played and continues to play in development of medical technologies and treatments. The problem lies in that small changes in the rate of funding growth lead to significant problems for individual researchers and their supporting institutions. These vicissitudes of waxing and waning funds mean ever-changing probabilities for securing peer-reviewed federal funding—a hopelessly unstable environment in which medical researchers are forced to work.

There is no single metric that serves as a surrogate to predict the appropriations process. As with any good evaluation, we will start with a good history and physical examination. The NIH has an important legislative and appropriations history. In addition to external forces, we will review the internal NIH priorities that continue to drive the funding process. Finally, we will end with a brief review of the impact congressionally mandated medical research programs have had on disease-specific funding.

A BRIEF HISTORY OF THE NATIONAL INSTITUTES OF HEALTH

There are key legislative events that have occurred in the past 80 years that have shaped the current form of the NIH. While their impact may seem distant and removed from the minutia of current day-to-day practices, they amply describe the current form and role the NIH plays in medical research

[a] Department of Urology, PenBay Medical Center, 3 Glen Cove Drive, Suite 3, Rockport, ME 04856, USA
[b] Department of Urology, Columbia-Presbyterian Hospital, College of Physicians and Surgeons, Columbia University, New York, NY, USA
* Corresponding author.
E-mail address: larsellison@gmail.com (L.M. Ellison).

Urol Clin N Am 36 (2009) 85–93
doi:10.1016/j.ucl.2008.08.008

funding. The NIH Web page provides a detailed outline of all related legislation.[3] The following is a synopsis of those elements that have profoundly effected funding for this governmental agency.

The NIH has its roots in the Marine Hospital Service (MHS). MHS was established in 1798 to care for sick and injured seamen. At that time, all seamen had a 20-cent per month deduction from their wages to fund the MHS. This forerunner of the Public Health Service continued unchanged until 1818 when the Navy developed its own medical service. Merchant marines remained covered under the MHS. During the 1800s, the primary authority of the MHS was monitoring for communicable disease outbreaks and initiation of quarantine as necessary.

In 1901, the first appropriation for a "hygienic laboratory" mandated "investigations of contagious and infectious diseases and matters pertaining to public health" (31 STAT. L. 1086).

In 1912, the name Public Health and Marine Hospital Service was changed to Public Health Service (PHS). This legislation broadened the PHS research program to include "diseases of man" and contributing factors such as pollution of navigable streams, and information dissemination (37 Stat. L. 309).

In 1931, the Ransdell Act reorganized, expanded, and renamed the Hygienic Laboratory as the National Institute of Health (P.L. 71-251, 46 Stat. L. 379).

In 1934, a law established the National Cancer Institute (NCI) to conduct and support research relating to the cause, diagnosis, and treatment of cancer. The law authorized the Surgeon General to make research grants in the field of cancer, provide fellowships, train personnel, and assist efforts in cancer prevention and control (P.L. 75-244, 50 Stat. L. 559).

In 1948, the National Heart Act created the National Heart Institute thus changing the name of National *Institute* of Health to National *Institutes* of Health (P.L. 80-655, 62 Stat. L. 464). With the creation of "institutes" under the umbrella of NIH, shifting political priorities and disease-specific interests came to increasingly dominate the appropriation process.

The year 1956 marked the first substantive investment in medical research facilities development. The Health Research Facilities Act (Title VII of the PHS act) authorized a PHS program of federal matching grants to public and nonprofit institutions for the construction of health research facilities (P.L. 84-835, 70 Stat. L. 717). With this act, the federal government became a major benefactor of hospital development by entering into the health systems construction business.

In 1960, a law amended the PHS act to authorize grants to universities, hospitals, laboratories, and other public and nonprofit institutions to strengthen their programs of research and research training health sciences (P.L. 86-798, 74 Stat. L. 1053). This act may be seen as the beginning of the modern federally funded research scientist.

In 1963 the Health Research Facilities Act of 1956 (Title VII to the PHS act) was revised to allow grants for multipurpose facilities that would provide teaching space as well as essential research space (P.L. 88-129, 77 Stat. L. 164). This program was extended in 1965 for construction of health research facilities (P.L. 89-115).

The Heart Disease, Cancer and Stroke Amendments of 1965 mandated regional cooperative programs in research, training, continuing education, and demonstration activities in patient care. The goal of integrating activities of medical schools, clinical research institutions and hospitals was to provide patients access to the latest treatment methods (P.L. 89-239).

1971, Congress passed into law the Supplemental Appropriations Bill, which included $100 million for cancer research. This appropriation was made in response to the President Nixon's State of the Union address, in which he called for "an intensive campaign to find a cure for cancer" (P.L. 92-18). The National Cancer Act of 1971 expanded the authority of NCI and NIH to advance research related to cancer. In addition, a National Cancer Advisory Board was established, and appropriations in excess of $400 million were authorized for FY1972 (P.L. 92-218). The National Cancer Act Amendments of 1974 authorized $2.5 billion over a 3-year period to extend and improve the National Cancer Program. Included in the language of the act was the following: establishment of the President's Biomedical Research Panel; provision for the President to appoint the director of NIH with the advice of the Senate; and requirement for peer review of NIH grant applications and contract projects (P.L. 93-352).

In 1980, the National Institute of Arthritis, Metabolism, and Digestive Diseases (NIAMDD) was renamed the National Institute of Arthritis, Diabetes, and Digestive and Kidney Diseases (NIDDK) (P.L. 96-538). The NIDDK and the NCI have been and continue to be the primary source for federal urologic research dollars.

The supplemental appropriations for FY 1983 provided funds for PHS AIDS activities. Specific line item earmarks included $9.4 million for NIH-directed AIDS research. This marked the first time the Congress directly appropriated money for AIDS research for NIH (P.L. 98-63). Through the 1980s, special interest groups gained increased traction regarding their abilities to guide and manipulate the federal appropriations process.

The budget of NIH was reduced in real terms under the Balanced Budget and Emergency Deficit Control Act of 1985 (Gramm-Rudman-Hollings). For NIH this reduction amounted to $236 million. The revised total NIH appropriation after Gramm-Rudman-Hollings became $5.3 billion, 4.3% below the original FY 1986 appropriation (P.L. 99-177).

In 1999, the grant submission process was significantly altered and streamlined. A common application was developed. In addition, the Mentored Clinical Scientist awards were developed and opened.

This select short list of pieces of legislation related to NIH is intended to highlight the transformation of the organization over the past century. What should be seen is that NIH has had its mandate shifted from a "public health" oversight organization to a research funding clearing house. The NIH has steadily been positioned to control and direct the trajectory of research endeavors in both the United States and other countries. The net effect of the transformation and the preeminence of NIH is a situation where medical researchers and many universities are intimately dependent on the stability and growth of the NIH budget.

MANAGEMENT OF THE GRANTING PROCESS

For the readership, it is likely well understood that most medical research projects are multiyear endeavors. The net result is that approximately 80% of the NIH budget for any given year is for ongoing projects. The remainder therefore is intended to cover new projects, 50% of which are investigator-initiated research project grants (RPG).[5,6] The pool of researchers competing for the limited NIH funds is a group of self-selected individuals who represent the best and the brightest among clinical and basic scientists. In the grant review process, proposals are reviewed, graded, and rank ordered based on scientific merit. What is clear is that, because of the high quality of the submissions, there becomes little difference among the top 30% to 40% of proposals. One NIH reviewer commented, "the ability to distinguish among a very small group of outstanding applications, which are the only ones that are going to get funded in the current climate, and to rank order then in any meaningful way is quite minimal."[7] As the threshold for funding begins to erode into the top cohort, the annual cumulative effect is a high rate of rejection and resubmission. While this competition may appear as

a healthy way to elevate of the quality of the pool, quite the contrary occurs. As the probability of funding declines, it does so in an asymmetric fashion. Those least likely to be funded are the junior researchers who have limited time to garner funding.[8] Most junior researchers will have departmental support for 2 to 3 years at which time they are expected to have secured the funding that moves them toward tenure-tract positions. Failure to obtain funding leads to an induced attrition of the younger cohort. These individuals often move toward the private sector. The alternative is to remain in a quasi postdoctoral position. Such a position means forced compromise in research agendas and thus diminished productivity; that very productivity that is necessary to ensure funding support in the future. In addition, senior-level researchers then support their junior colleagues for longer periods of time. For an institution, reduced numbers of grants translates to lower revenues. Thus the net effect is an ever-larger financial burden for research shifted from the federal government to public and private academic institutions.

In an elegant study, Korn and colleagues[6] modeled growth patterns for NIH and their impact on medical research. The motivation for their study related to anticipated changes in appropriations following a rapid period of growth of the NIH budget between 1998 and 2003. Among the principals they prioritized were preservation of the integrity and merit of the peer-review process, maintenance of new investigators, sustaining commitments to ongoing awards, preservation of the capacity of awardee institutions, recognition of the need of contemporary biomedical science, and maintenance of the intramural NIH program. To ensure stability of these elements, the authors measured capacity at a series of appropriation growth rates. They found 8% to 9% growth led to a stable 32% success of securing funding for projects. A 4% NIH appropriation growth rate leads to a substantial deceleration of grant submissions and funding success. The authors did not model growth below 4% because "the tradeoffs and sacrifices that would have been caused... were too difficult to deal with in the model."

MACROECONOMIC TRENDS
EFFECTING APPROPRIATIONS

Over the past 35 years, there have been occasions when the growth of the final approved NIH budget grew by less than 4% from the prior year (**Fig. 1**). Four of those eight occasions have occurred since 2003. What is more, no prior occurrence was more

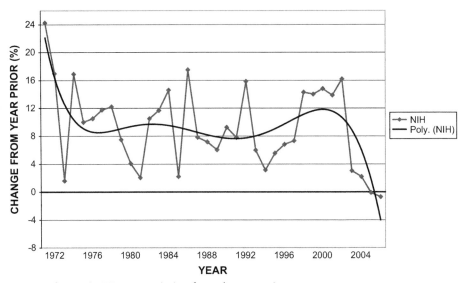

Fig. 1. Percentage change in NIH appropriation from the year prior.

than a single year anomaly. A look back at the four prior occurrences may provide insight into forces at play more recently.

In 1974, the economy of the United States was reeling from the Saudi oil embargo. Significant cuts in budgetary items were noted across all domestic spending. As a result, even the new-found enthusiasm for the "War on Cancer" had little capacity to counteract the prevailing economic downturn. The budget for NIH rose from $1.76 billion in 1973 to $1.79 billion in 1974. The loss of momentum was short lived. In 1975, the NIH budget grew by 16% to $2.10 billion and an additional 9% in 1976 to $2.30 billion.

In 1982, then President Regan was focused on reducing a very real and ballooning of the domestic budget. NIH appropriations grew by 2% in 1982 from $3.57 billion to $3.64 billion. Just as in 1974, the flat growth rate of funding was short lived. In the subsequent 3 years the budget at NIH grew by 10.5%, 11.5%, and 14.6% respectively, to $5.15 billion in 1985.

In 1985, Gramm-Rudman-Hollings Balanced Budget Act mandated a reduction in deficit spending to 0% within 5 years.[9] This across-the-board legislation resulted in a 2% growth of the budget to $5.26 billion. Just as with prior episodes of budgetary constraint, the following year, 1986, NIH received a 17% increase in appropriations to $6.18 billion.

In 1994, the first midterm election for President Clinton, the Republican Party introduced a significant challenge in the form of the "Contract With America." Among the eight points listed in the contract was a pledge for fiscal responsibility in the form of a balanced budget. The 1995 NIH budget was $11.3 billion, just 3% over that of 1994. Just as with the prior flattening in the rate of growth, the subsequent years saw healthy rises of 5.6%, 6.8%, and 7.3%.

THE DOUBLING ERA

Between 1998 and 2003 the NIH budget grew from $14 billion to $28 billion. This concerted effort on the part of the federal government was the largest and most rapid growth in the history of NIH.[5] It is important to realize that this did not simply represent five consecutive benevolent years. Rather, this effort was planned and orchestrated to push medical research at a time when technologies and the human genome project were on the brink of producing substantial returns on investment. In response to this federal initiative, medical schools developed infrastructure, hired new faculty, and developed new training programs.

The rate of spending at medical schools has grown exponentially in the past 20 years. Spending increased from $2.2 billion to $3.9 billion to $7.4 billion for the periods 1990 to 1997, 1998 to 2002, and 2003 to 2007, respectively.[7] While there are certainly other elements at play in the expansion and development of medical school campuses (expansion of the MD workforce as a major contributor), the preeminent role of federally funded research cannot be overlooked. That new capacity required active physicians and researchers. For some institutions, there has been a rise of faculty numbers that approaches 50%.

The real impact of the changing NIH appropriations was felt at the researcher level. Between 1998 and 2007 the number of scientists submitting

RPGs grew by 75% from 20,000 to upwards of 35,000.[10] For the 1998 to 2003 period, the budget growth allowed for stable overall rates of funded proposals at the 30% level. The numbers of applicants continued to rise after 2003. The flattening NIH budget then resulted in a steep drop off in funding levels to below 20%. For NCI the approval rate for funding was just 11% in 2006, down from 16% in 2005.[11]

This picture is even bleaker for the most junior researchers. For those individuals just out of training, the overall probability of securing NIH funding was just 9% in 2006. This was down from near parity with the established researcher cohort as recently as 2001. The average age for securing NIH funding was 42 years old in 2006.[12] This is up from 35 years old in 1970. While disturbing, there is increased cause for worry as this relates data on cumulative career productivity. It has been shown that innovations in biomedical research come from young researchers in their 30s; the group most likely to fail to secure grant funding.[13]

The belt tightening required at NIH has significant impact for funded researchers. The most striking and overt is a new policy at NCI that in effect states that approved projects will receive 29% less money than requested.[11] Certainly, this may allow for more projects to be funded, but the trickle down to the researcher is substantial. A project budget that is cut by nearly one third may not be able to support the expected involvement of a postdoctoral or graduate student; or elements of the research plan may not be feasible. Alternatively, the administrative dollars collected by the supporting university may be reduced, thus requiring unanticipated additional cost sharing.

While the Doubling Era was a heady and exciting time, it was quite clear that the levels of growth could not be sustained, and therefore a new "post-doubling" policy toward NIH appropriations would need to be developed. That plan however was absent, and what is more, geopolitical issues (Iraq/Afghanistan War, Katrina, and escalating energy prices) have served to undercut appropriations to a much greater extent than anticipated.

The absolute erosion of appropriations has been quite startling over the past 3 years (**Fig. 1**).[1,14] Most striking is that in 2006 to 2007, the NIH budget actually shrank by 1.1% and then 1.8%. This is the first year that there has been an actual drop in the NIH budget. Not only is the appropriation failing to meet minimal standards to support its prior mission (8% growth), it is failing to keep pace with biomedical research inflation calculated at 3.7%. This would be a stark and concerning situation if it did not follow 2 prior years of 3.0% and 2.2% growth respectively. In effect, the current administration is dismantling the capacity created during the prior 8-year expansion of NIH.

CONGRESSIONALLY DIRECTED MEDICAL RESEARCH PROGRAMS

The Congressionally Directed Medical Research Program (CDMRP) is a constellation of earmarked appropriations for specific disease entities. These are clearly important initiatives. The problem with these "mandates" is that the recipient of the mandate is taking finite dollars that would have been distributed in peer-review manner at the institute level. To be sure, urology has been a beneficiary of this program, primarily in the form of prostate cancer research.

There is a long and contentious history associated with the allocation of federal funds for cancer research. Much of the controversy arose in the early 1990s. With impending budgetary constraint, advocacy groups increasingly lobbied congressional offices and NIH for more research on their specific disease of interest. These efforts succeeded for certain diseases (eg, AIDS and breast cancer) at the expense of others. Limited budget resources added to the intensity of fierce lobbying for disease-specific mandates in the NIH budget. As a result of the continuing controversy over disease funding, congressional hearings were held in 1997 addressing the mechanisms for establishing research priorities at NIH.

As an example of the impact of disproportional funding related to disease incidence, the following describes federal funding for AIDS research for 1998 and 1999: "For FY1998, NIH is allocating a total of $1.61 billion for AIDS research, or 12% of the $13.6 billion total NIH budget. Funding for research on AIDS in FY1998 is second only to the National Cancer Institute ($2.3 billion). Government-wide AIDS spending is estimated at $9.67 billion in FY1999."[15] The funding for HIV/AIDS remains stable at 10.2% of the NIH budget for the years 2003 to 2007.

The allocation for AIDS research is startling in its magnitude. Furthermore, if examined in light of disease prevalence and mortality, the level of funding is even more disproportionate. Overall, there were a total of 566,000 reported cases of AIDS and 340,000 AIDS-related deaths in the United States between the years 1980 and 1996.[16] In contrast, there were 1,359,000 new cancer cases and 554,000 cancer-related deaths in the United States in 1996 alone. There are twice as many incident cases of cancer and 60% more cancer deaths in the single year 1996 than occurred as a result of AIDS during the entire epidemic from 1980 to 1996.

Prostate cancer research funding by NCI has significantly increased since 1998. In the early 1990s, the annual allocation grew from $13 million in 1990 to $71 million in 1996.[17] Even with these increases, the 1996 funding level for prostate cancer ranked among the lowest four cancers by incidence. However, with mandates from Congress to expand funding of prostate (and breast cancer), the levels continued to rise. Allocations rose to $135.7 million in 1999 and $203.2 million in 2000. By 2000, prostate cancer funding was second only to breast cancer ($438.7 million). For the years 2003 to 2007, the allocated funds for prostate cancer research ranged from a high of $379 million to $347 million most recently. As demonstrated above, the use of absolute allocations as the measure of funding parity, while interesting, do not account for differences in disease impact on society. While federal support of prostate cancer research rose dramatically in the late 1990s, there remain disparities in allocations when examined in relation to various epidemiologic measures.

Incidence rates may be used as a weight to adjust absolute levels of allocation. In other words, we could look at dollars per incident case of cancer. In 2007, there were 218,890 new cases of prostate cancer in the United States. Second was lung and bronchus cancer, with 213,380 new cases; and third was breast cancer with 180,510. The rise in absolute appropriations might at first glance lead one to believe the current distribution of funds is reasonable. However, funding levels are adjusted for incidence, we find that in 2000, prostate cancer ranks 11th behind Hodgkin's disease and just above lung and bronchus cancer (**Fig. 2**).

Alternatively, annual disease-specific mortality could be the measure upon which allocations are adjusted. In 2000, the prostate cancer–related death rate ranked fourth behind lung, colon, and breast cancer at 31,900 deaths/year. When adjusting appropriations based on mortality rate, prostate cancer ranks sixth behind leukemia (**Fig. 3**). What is more, while breast cancer ranks second after this adjustment, colon cancer ranks 10th and lung and bronchus cancer ranks 14th.

Clearly the decision process influencing allocation of funds is driven by a number of "hard" and "soft" variables. Among the hard variables, health-services researchers have examined, as above, the ability of incidence and mortality as well as years of life lost and prevalence to predict appropriations. No single crude epidemiologic measure sufficiently describes the relationship.[18] Presumably a complex model weighting each variable would approximate the process. Gross and colleagues[19] examined NIH budget requests for 1996 in relation to incidence, prevalence, mortality, and disability-adjusted life-years (DALYs). The DALY is a downward adjustment of the value of a year of life with a specific disability relative to no disability. Of the four measures, the authors found a significant relationship between NIH funding and DALYs. However, the prediction model accompanying this analysis accounted for only 62% of the variability of funding by disease. Therefore, the interplay of incidence, prevalence, and mortality, as well as the efforts of the numerous lobbying groups on Capital Hill also influenced the process.

While there has never been a full disclosure of the methods used, NCI/NIH has publicly

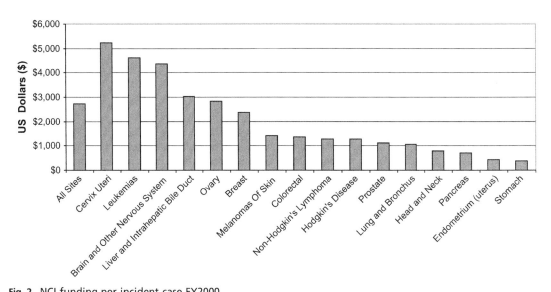

Fig. 2. NCI funding per incident case FY2000.

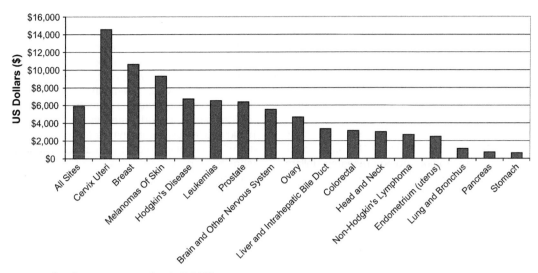

Fig. 3. NCI funding per cancer death FY2000.

acknowledged the above debates.[20] In response, they identify several constraints within the process that limit the flexibility for and speed of change. First, for any given year, 80% of the budget is allocated to continuation of multiyear projects. Second, they identify the need for rapid response to unforeseen public health needs (ie, Ebola virus, smallpox and anthrax investigations). Finally, it is suggested that many research activities, while assigned to a given disease, will generate findings that translate to and inform other disease processes.

What is the value of weighting allocations? A bar for assisting to determine the level of federal funding for research for a given disease is nonexistent. Superficially there appears to be a rank order to determining funding levels. However, when the system fails to demonstrate logical consistency, it can only follow that external forces have distorted the process to their own ends. In this case, it is clear that the special interest groups that have come to play such an important role on Capital Hill have negatively impacted the distribution of federal funds. The above examples, using incidence and mortality as weighting systems, allow for simple calculation of funding levels based on known and accepted epidemiologic measures.

Politics are intertwined with health care policy and funding. While this is not a new phenomenon, the level of interaction is unprecedented and growing. The "War on Cancer" has been waged for close to 35 years, and significant strides have been made. In the past 15 years the determination of funding allocation has been adversely influenced by special interest groups. Given that lobbying has de facto been legislated, to its credit

the American Urological Association (AUA) has been effective in advancing prostate cancer as a significant agenda item within NCI.

Although prostate cancer has benefited from funding trends in the past decade, there remain casualties of the funding process in urological cancer: kidney cancer and bladder cancer. Together kidney cancer and bladder cancer accounted for nearly 87,000 new cancer cases and 25,000 cancer deaths in 2000.[17] Compared with lymphomas or leukemias, kidney and bladder cancer have higher rates of incidence and mortality. The funding levels for these sites are not included as a line item in the published annual budget submitted to Congress. However, NIH does report its ongoing research portfolio by cancer site.[21] As a crude comparison, there are currently 1628 funded studies of lymphoma and 1043 funded studies of leukemia. The NCI currently reports 395 funded studies of kidney cancer and 333 funded studies of bladder cancer. As a comparison, there are 1183 currently funded studies of prostate cancer and 2037 funded studies for breast cancer. With recent approvals for new first-line therapy for metastatic kidney cancer and studies suggesting a rise in the incidence of kidney cancer, it would certainly seem prudent for NCI to identify this as an area of particular interest, as well as address the apparent deficiency in bladder cancer research funding.

THE AMERICAN UROLOGICAL ASSOCIATION AS ADVOCATE FOR UROLOGY RESEARCH FUNDING

The era of the physician-scientist may be coming to a close. For many young MDs, the chances for

NIH funding have been substantially eroded in recent years. As noted in prior sections, the competition for declining federal research dollars is all the more problematic given the rising numbers of applicants for RO1 and other mechanisms. With increased competition, MD is quite simply less capable of competing with PhD, particularly in the field of basic science.

The AUA has made substantial efforts to interface with the various institutes at NIH so as to advocate for ever-eroding urology research dollars. The NIDDK has traditionally been the primary source (outside of NCI) for urology funding. Even these efforts have failed to thwart an increasing shift in the NIDDK portfolio toward nephrology-related projects. Recent comments from the acting director of the NIDDK, "established investigators are leaving the field (of urology research), and young investigators are not attracted to it," seem to stand in stark contrast to the ever-increasing size of academic departments at the major training institutions.[22] It is quite disheartening and appears somewhat self-serving, that our nephrology colleagues would make such claims without providing supporting objective data. However, in fairness, the acting director then went on in the same article to discuss the potential pathways to enhance the competitiveness of urology in the NIH granting system.

The AUA has established a program to assist the physician-scientist. It is recognized that the balance of research (essentially unpaid labor) and clinical practice leads to a very difficult financial balance not only for individuals but their supporting departments. The K award mechanism, a training grant to help individuals on the path to an RO1, has required a 75% time commitment to research. As surgeons this becomes an untenable situation. The AUA has successfully negotiated a revised commitment down from 75% to 50%. In addition, the AUA established a supplemental funding program. Under this AUA-NIH Surgeon Scientist Award, the recipient would receive supplemental salary support for the duration of the award for up to 5 years. The amount of support has a scheduled increase annually beginning at $28,000 the first year to $52,000 the fifth year. Each year two recipients will be selected from the applicant pool. More information is available at www2.niddk.nih.gov/Funding/TrainingCareerDev.

SUMMARY

The future of federal appropriations for NIH is in a period of significant and possibly catastrophic downturn. There has never been a sustained flattening let alone reduction in funding levels of the proportion seen in the past 5 years. There are certainly budgetary constraints with the wars in Iraq and Afghanistan and the necessary redirection of funds toward military support. As a nation we are clearly in the throws of attempting to find common ground between our various diametrically opposed political camps. Unfortunately in the process, the medical research community is feeling a "perfect storm" of negative forces: increasing institutional capacity, increasing numbers of medical researchers, diminishing appropriated funds, and geopolitical pressures with no evidence of abatement. We must as a nation continue to commit ourselves to research and development. Our strength and our preeminence in the world are dependent on a vibrant and progressive scientific community. One can only hope that the wisdom of the legislature and the executive branches will see the critical importance that NIH plays in maintaining our position in the global economy, and make the appropriate decisions related to medical research funding.

REFERENCES

1. Appropriations for the National Institutes of Health, Fiscal Year 2007. Office of Legislative Policy and Analysis. Available at: http://olpa.od.nih.gov/legislation/109/pendinglegislation/approp2007.asp. Accessed May 2, 2007.
2. Porter J. Federal funding and supportive policies for research. JAMA 2005;294(11):1385–9.
3. Nih. Almanac: historical data. NIH. Available at: http://history.nih.gov/01Docs/historical/LegislativeChronologyLaws.htm. Accessed May 30, 2007.
4. Loscalzo J. The NIH budget and the future of biomedical research. N Engl J Med 2006;354(16):1665–7.
5. Zerhouni E. NIH in the post-doubling era: realities and strategies. Science 2006;314:1088–90.
6. Korn D, Rich R, Garrison H, et al. The NIH in the "Postdoubling" era. Science 2002;296:1401–2.
7. Couzin J, Miller G. Boom and bust. Science 2007; 316:356–61.
8. Marks A. Rescuing the NIH before it is too late. J Clin Invest 2006;116(4):844.
9. Gramm-Rudman-Hollings Balanced Budget and Emergency Deficit Control Act of 1985. (Pub.L. 99–177, title II, December 12, 1985, 99 Stat. 1038, 2 U.S.C. § 900).
10. Mandel H, Vessell E. From progress to regression: biomedical research funding. J Clin Invest 2004; 114(7):872–6.
11. Finkelstein J. NIH and related agencies face a flat budget future. J Natl Cancer Inst 2006;98(6): 376–7.

12. Weinberg R. A lost generation. Cell 2006;126: 9–10.

13. Vastag B. Increasing RO1 competition concerns researchers. J Natl Cancer Inst 2006;98(20):1436–8.

14. Appropriations for the National Insititutes of Health, Fiscal year 2006. Office of legislative policy and analysis. Available at: http://olpa.od.nih.gov/legislation/109/pendinglegislation/approp2006.asp. Accessed March 27, 2007.

15. Johnson JA. AIDS funding for federal government programs: FY1981–FY1999. Washington, DC: Congressional Research Service Science, Technology, and Medicine Division Library of Congress; 1998.

16. Kirschstein R. Disease-specific estimates of direct and indirect costs of illness and NIH support. Washington, DC: Department of Health and Human Services; 2000. P. HR106–370.

17. The 2002 NCI Budget Request. National Cancer Institute 10/12/2001. Available at: http://2002.cancer.gov/2002.htm. Accessed June 15, 2007.

18. Michaud C, Murray C, Bloom B. Burden of disease: implications for future research. JAMA 2001;285(5): 535–9.

19. Gross CP, Anderson GF, Powe NR. The relation between funding by the National Institutes of Health and the burden of disease. N Engl J Med 1999; 340(24):1881–7.

20. Setting WGoP. Setting research priorities at the National Institutes of Health. Washington, DC: National Instutites of Health; 1997.

21. NIH Research Portfolio. NIH. Available at: www.researchportfolio.cancer.gov. Accessed June 15, 2007.

22. Star R. Advancing urology research: NIDDK and AUA team to effect change. AUA News 2007.

Supergroups and Economies of Scale

Steven Schlossberg, MD, MBA[a,b,c],*

KEYWORDS
• Merger activity • Organizational goals and structure
• Economies of scale

Over the last several years, there has been an increasing consolidation of physician practices in general, and urology has been no exception. Although many of these consolidations or mergers have been between two small practices, others have involved the creation of previously not seen urology groups covering large geographic areas as the result of a merger of many practices. These "supergroups" have varied from in size from 20 to 50 urologists. What defines a supergroup? The simple definition may be a group of urologists who can expand the line of services well beyond traditional urologic practice. These groups create value in two large categories: horizontal and vertical integration. Horizontal integration combines existing practices in the activities of traditional physician practice. Vertical integration refers to the addition of services to customers that are likely a natural extension of the conventional activities.

What are economies of scale? In simple economic terms, the term means a decreasing cost of production as the number of units made increases. It also can refer to the decreasing cost of an activity as the scale of an activity (ie, marketing or distribution) increases. Does the formation of supergroups produce economies of scale? Is that the reason to merge practices? If not, what is the value proposition? If so, how often are groups successful? Why has this activity increased significantly over the last 5 years?

By way of introduction, advising physicians to merge for economies of scale in a true economic sense is wrong. The prize is not cutting overhead the way a physician might traditionally think but improving management and enhancing revenue.

Typically the model is to merge practices into a single entity, but physicians often do not consolidate their offices. There are areas in which money can be saved: sharing a management information system, electronic medical records (EMRs), or administrator at a level that each group could not afford individually. These are economies of scale, but most physicians think of economies of scale as overall cost reductions. Overall, total costs generally go up but the benefits from these cost increases come from improved billing and collection performance, coding, better management of personnel, human resources, HIPPA compliance, and information technology.

Increased size strengthens the group practice's negotiating position with hospitals, employers, insurance companies, managed care organizations, and other third-party payers. This development may enable a physician to participate with a third-party payer who had not even considered contracting with the physician or smaller group before the practice merger. As information related to patient satisfaction, peer review, quality assurance, and use management becomes more important, practices that have these data available have a better chance of succeeding. This also makes the merged group more attractive to such payers, possibly enabling physicians to obtain better payment rates than they received before the merger. Forming a larger group practice enables merged practices to maintain or strengthen their market share in the area. The merged practice is able to offer more full-service care and greater continuity of care for patients. The size of a larger group enables the physicians within the practice to

a Department of Urology, Eastern Virginia Medical School, Norfolk, VA, USA
b Department of Medical Informatics, Sentara Healthcare, Norfolk, VA, USA
c Health Policy, American Urologic Association, Linthicum, MD, USA
* 6333 Center Drive, Norfolk, VA 23502.
E-mail address: smschlos@sentara.com

Urol Clin N Am 36 (2009) 95–100
doi:10.1016/j.ucl.2008.08.002

provide better coverage for one another in a more cost-efficient manner. The resources that a larger group possesses may allow the physicians within the merged group to attain goals and advance their practices beyond what would have been attainable before the merger. The increased financial resources of the group may allow the group to purchase major medical equipment, recruit greater expertise in management, offer additional ancillary services, and recruit additional physicians.

This article covers the following topics and elaborates on the general thoughts mentioned previously:

- External forces driving mergers
- Organizational goals and structure
- Categories of economies of scale
  - Business operational activities
  - Horizontal integration
  - Resources and knowledge
  - Information technology and quality improvement
  - Vertical integration

WHAT ARE THE EXTERNAL FORCES DRIVING MERGER ACTIVITY?

To most practicing physicians, the answer to this question is apparent. Urologists may differ, however, as to which of the many forces is the most important to encourage merger for their group or them personally. I discuss these drivers in no specific order, but all have been cited as a reason for this activity.

Decreasing reimbursement from the federal government is clearly one of the primary drivers. Over the last 5 years, physicians essentially have seen no increase in payments, which turns to a negative because expenses continue to rise. Commercial rates are often pegged to federal (Medicare) reimbursement. Several years ago, physicians also experienced a decrease in reimbursement for pharmaceutical purchases and dispensing of in-office medications for chemotherapy, taking away a source of profit that subsidized complicated cancer care. Third-party commercial reimbursement trends have varied depending on region of the country, so it is hard to make any sweeping statements.

For urologists, a second important driver has been the manpower shortage: it is difficult to recruit new partners. This shortage has been created by the surge in demand from the aging of the population and our different practice patterns. New diagnostic tests and new treatments for old problems have increased the workload for urologists. Two simple examples are (1) the increasing number of radical prostatectomies being done currently compared with 10 to 15 years ago with the increase in prostate-specific antigen testing and (2) the increase in female incontinence procedures with improvements in results and patient morbidity. Finally, some speculate that because of the increase in "hassle factor" of practice, physicians are retiring earlier.

A third driver is the increasing complexity of urologic practice from a business and clinical perspective. On the business side, physicians have tried to improve the running of their practices by becoming more involved. This task has become more difficult, however, in the setting of the increasing burden of keeping up with federal and third-party contracting issues, the "alphabet soup" of unfunded mandates from regulations (ie, HIPPAA and others), and the need for information technology in a background of flat reimbursement and the physician's desire to do more clinically. On the clinical side, the definition of a full-service urologic practice has changed with the trend to subspecialization either after fellowship training or based on area of interest; most physicians realize it is hard to be good at everything! With subspecialization, many physicians prefer to have a colleague who also subspecializes—an additional driver to a larger size.

Fourth, physicians from all specialties—especially urologists—have realized the practice benefit of vertical integration. With flat reimbursement and increasing inefficiencies at many hospitals secondary to their own problems, many urologists try to avoid going to the hospital unless absolutely necessary. Simply said, they are much more efficient in their own offices, and because of improvements in treatment options, more procedures can be done through office-based or medical-based therapies.

Finally, I often ask physicians if, knowing what they know about medical practice today, they would create a model of a one- or two-person group. Although not universal, most people say that the status quo is not sustainable without some significant changes to scope of practice or income.

ORGANIZATIONAL GOALS AND STRUCTURE

Over the years, many different legal structures have been discussed as alternatives to complete merger. Although a detailed discussion is beyond the scope of this article, large groups usually create one legal entity with consolidated business operations and different operating divisions. Ultimately, the correct structure accomplishes a balance to allow the discipline for developing and implementing a group strategy while preserving appropriate physician or divisional autonomy. In other words, centralize what adds value but leave flexibility for local decisions that do not affect the entire group. To further explain these thoughts, some examples may help.

Because compensation is a way to drive behavior, many groups leave physician compensation to the divisional structure. Often, some significant percentage might be tied to individual productivity. Any compensation derived from central services such as imaging or laboratory testing is often divided based on number of physicians rather than referral volume, however. To be successful, programmatic development should occur with a group perspective in mind. As the program is implemented, many divisional issues may occur around logistics, such as schedules and operational support by divisional staff. All parts of the large group need to work together to ensure success rather than evolve into blaming "them" for the problem. In this situation, "them" is actually "us." Finally, what about implementing an EMR? This is clearly a group decision that affects divisional operations. To be successful, all physicians need to meet a minimum standard of adoption so that the group can achieve their objectives likely around quality of care and cost savings to pay for the implementation.

What about economies of scale? Can an organizational structure support this premise? The answer is yes. With more physicians supporting a central structure, the group can decide which services it wants to bring inside versus what services it wants to outsource. For example, do you need a chief financial officer? Should you have a bookkeeper and have an accounting firm on retainer? The latter construct is a good example of employing the less expensive worker who is doing a significant amount of work and having a contract with the higher priced expertise, the certified public accountant whose time is needed on a more limited basis. Cost comes from underemploying an expensive resource; however, employing a group of certified medical coders who work in your central business office is a good example of a valuable in-house service. What about an administrator? A larger group can afford a more sophisticated, experienced, and professional manager who can more than pay for the position and not cost more on a per physician basis than the cost for a less experienced person in a smaller group. The person easily pays for the position through managing the many issues that develop as a larger group forms, develops, and refines a strategy in the ever-changing health care environment.

CATEGORIES OF ECONOMIES OF SCALE
Business Operational Activities

In this category, one should consider all the functions to make the practice run. These issues span the topic of human resources to insurance contracting to the billing office. All three of these topics have become more complex over time. The topics of knowledgeable resources and information technology are addressed subsequently in other sections.

The human resource function has become increasingly important for practices as they try to create leverage of physician's time, automate functions, and maintain a work force. Because training and education require an investment of time, a larger practice can devote resources to develop a training program for employees. Like many topics, this investment of time becomes more affordable as the cost is spread over many employees. If physicians are to do what they are uniquely qualified to do to maintain income, then it is essential to develop, maintain, and grow this function. As part of recruitment and retention, benefits management is also a critical function. A larger group can devote more time or contract for more sophisticated expertise to get the most value for the dollars spent on this process. The employment of physician extenders is a great example of economies of scale. Although initially physicians say, "Let's hire a nurse practitioner to become more efficient," appropriate hiring and use is not a trivial task. What is the right ratio of extender to physician? How do you bill? What is their scope of practice? How do you train? Like many topics, it is easier to hire a third nurse practitioner because much of the work is done after the first two are in place.

Insurance contracting is an example of work that needs to be done whether you are a 5-, 10-, or 15-person physician practice. It is critical to have the expertise and track your information to understand the many nuances of this process. A detailed explanation is beyond the scope of this article, but ask yourself this question: Is a small group able to afford the same amount of time as a large group to do a detailed analysis of each payor contract and payment policies? Similar observations can be made about your billing system. Although some practices choose to outsource this function to a third party, someone within the practice needs to review, manage, and hold this third party accountable. Charge entry and delinquent claims often fall to practice resources.

Horizontal Integration

This term refers to the merging of existing practices to reduce duplication and achieve efficiencies. In this context, the topic is usually clinical practice. There are some clear-cut winners where duplication can be reduced: (1) better call coverage at hospitals, (2) merging and closing offices to rationalize capacity, (3) clinical referrals that promote quality and allow specialization of clinical service, and (4) less duplication of basic diagnostic equipment. During strategic planning, this is a topic that clearly needs to be addressed. Results may be difficult to achieve initially, however. The conversation may bring out old areas of conflict between senior partners; something less seen recently. The consultants approach this by harvesting the "low hanging fruit." Do what is simple and can be achieved easily. Do not overreach. Achieve some successes to create credibility. The successful groups then build on their achievements to take on the harder tasks over time. This may be a 3- to 5-year process to achieve complete integration of existing practices.

Do these economies of scale have a payback? Is it economic? When a practice can achieve better use of a fixed cost (rent for office), the economics improve. What are the economies of scale for a better call schedule? Can practices decide which physicians work at which hospitals? "Does everyone have to go everywhere?" It clearly creates value that may not have a measurable economic benefit other than if some efficiencies of practice can be achieved.

Resources and Knowledge

With any knowledge worker, it is nice to have a critical mass of people who can share, understand, and process their ever-changing field. These thoughts can be extended to all levels of workers—from the front desk clerks to the office managers to the physicians. It is clearly true of physicians. In a work environment, it is more attractive to be one of three urologic oncologists than the only one in a group. The same applies to physician extenders and certified coders. Although obvious when stated, this is something that is usually not discussed until groups are created and operational. The groups that are through the initial start-up process of merging cultures clearly realize this as a significant benefit.

Information Technology and Quality Improvement

Although many groups merge for various reasons, EMRs and quality improvement are not usually their top reasons. In fact, significant economies can be achieved in these areas with scale. The conversation can certainly be one of "make" versus "buy," but the physician practice needs to do a significant amount of work to achieve success in these areas. An EMR will be the foundation of the physician practice over the next several years. Although most quality programs rely on reporting of measures through the billing system (ie, Medicare physician quality reporting initiative), data capture at the point of care in an EMR will be a benefit in several years and become essential in the long-term.

Implementing an EMR for a practice can be a daunting task. Often what happens falls into one of three approaches: no decision because of cost and complexity, a decision to move forward laced with many unforeseen events that alter success ("They didn't know what they didn't know"), or—in the minority—a well thought out and successful implementation. What does it take to be successful and how do economies of scale help?

EMR implementation requires many labor-intensive efforts and a fair amount of expertise. Although many practices may be purchasing their second billing system, few, if any, are purchasing their second EMR. The factors that drive most results relate to the lack of experience and implications of a bad decision. To start, practices need to develop criteria and evaluate potential vendors: a request for proposal process. Some practices may engage a consultant, whereas others try to do it in-house. This process needs to be done once whether it is a 5-person group or a 25-person group. With all the evaluation costs, this should be a fixed, one-time expense that can be spread over the larger number of physicians. The real savings come from ongoing costs, application improvement, and equipment maintenance.

Ongoing costs for an EMR can be divided into certain fixed and variable costs. The following discussion refers to a system owned and maintained by the practice. If a practice chooses a remote computing or application service provider approach, then the costs tend to be fixed, but on a per-user basis. Depending on the vendor, with a larger practice and appropriate length of contract, they may amortize the cost of startup into the monthly fee. A larger number of users confers economic benefit to the practice. If a practice decides to own and maintain the application, then true fixed and variable costs are incurred. The fixed costs are incurred in a step function. For example, when purchasing the main hardware, often it is sized for a group of users so that the cost per user goes down as the number of users increases. The personnel to maintain and manage the infrastructure also tends to be a fixed cost, but it is helpful to develop a critical mass of people for redundancy of support and from a knowledge perspective. There are many different configurations for the support of the application and network services. One generalization clearly is true: whether dealing with a company and a purchase or outsourcing some of the support of an in-house application (ie, network services), a better price on a per-physician basis is obtained by the larger group.

The second category of benefit size confers is content management for the users. Many EMRs come with preconfigured content that is often customized for a specialty. One of the key drivers of success for an EMR implementation is customized training for workflow and content for the specialty, however. Being able to get 3 or 4 physicians together who can then help a larger group of 20 physicians is another way to achieve economies of scale. These physicians focus on how to adapt the software product to the specialty specific content and the way the practice would treat patients using this new tool. Without this initial, significant investment of time, many EMR installations in the past have just automated the old and not achieved the proposed benefit or point-of-care documentation for the physicians.

In a similar way, a larger group is likely able to track and implement the many quality initiatives that are just starting to become requirements of practice. Currently, most of these initiatives are tracked through claims submission. In the future, the EMR will help practices collect these at the point of care. The data can be harvested and submitted as needed based on contracts and requirements. Scale helps in two ways: (1) the process needs to be designed once for 5 or 20 physicians, and (2) the application of physician time to develop it and incorporate it into the practice can be done by a few to help the larger group.

Vertical Integration

Physicians often have incorporated things into their practice to facilitate the immediate care of patients. Many years ago, in-office laboratories made things easier for primary care physicians. Routine radiographic equipment is often part of primary care or specialist practices. For years, multispecialty groups have offered many services beyond the traditional single-specialty practice, such as ambulatory surgery centers and more complicated imaging centers. With the development of larger single specialty groups, vertical integration refers to developing a center in which most outpatient services performed by the urologist occur within a facility owned and managed by the practice. Other ancillary services may be provided. This trend started approximately 10 to 15 years ago and recently has become increasingly more prevalent. Several factors have driven this trend, including the shift of urologic practice from inpatient to outpatient services, the decreasing cost of some of the diagnostic and therapeutic modalities, convenience of care delivery for the physician and patient, perception by patients and physicians that "I would rather not go to the hospital if I did not have to go," and profitability of these services. Although smaller practices have done some of these things, the larger groups have done all of them starting 10 years ago, only limited by some state legislation around certificate of need programs. These are state-specific programs that limit who can own certain health care facilities and equipment. Typically, this legislation focuses on ambulatory surgery centers, expensive diagnostic equipment (ie, CT and MRI), and therapeutic modalities (ie, radiation therapy).

In terms of vertical integration, many of the comments regarding other initiatives are true for these programs. The list is variable but typically includes ambulatory surgery center, CT scan, urodynamic testing, pathology, physical therapy, and, more recently, radiation therapy. Some of these programs typically are different as to why a large group can extend its services to include these programs. Expertise and specialization are two reasons why super groups confer economies of scale. In this situation, specialty support staff can be developed and maintained to increase quality and efficiency. With urodynamics, a specially trained nurse or technician can perform these studies on a routine basis. With the prevalence of voiding dysfunction, many large groups can support two people who do nothing but urodynamic testing with physician supervision. Because they become facile at setup, performance, and interpretation, physicians can supervise the key parts of the procedure but ultimately do what they are uniquely qualified to do. Similarly, some groups have been able to hire a physical therapist who does nothing but pelvic floor exercises. The therapist can provide a valuable service to patients with various urologic conditions. As with urodynamic testing, the quality of care is often better than can be obtained through hospital services.

Pathology and imaging services provide a combination of true economies of scale and concentration of expertise with improvement in understanding of the disease being diagnosed. Any large group can easily support an in-house pathology laboratory and imaging center, which provides a convenience factor for patients and physicians. Some groups have hired radiologists and pathologists as partners to obtain reliable and constant readings. Dedicated services from colleagues who perform ancillary interpretation are widely recognized to produce more consistent and accurate readings. Others choose to contract with local physicians to perform the professional service component of this testing.

With all these services, the large groups have no problem supporting the economics of this approach. Recently, regulators have been concerned about overuse of physician-owned ancillary services, especially in the context of the Medicare population. For the many reasons discussed previously, the large groups have no problem providing quality service and supporting their economic investment. More importantly, this integrated approach to urologic care provides better and more convenient care for the Medicare population.

SUMMARY

With the changing environment for medical practice, physician practice models will continue to evolve. These "supergoups" create economies of scale, but their advantage is not only in the traditional economic sense. Practices with enough size are able to better meet the challenges of medical practice with increasing regulatory demands, explosion of clinical knowledge, quality and information technology initiatives, and an increasingly tight labor market. Smaller practices can adapt some of these strategies selectively. Depending on the topic, smaller practices should think differently about how to approach the challenges of practice.

Medical Malpractice: The Good, the Bad, and the Ugly

Kevin R. Loughlin, MD, MBA

KEYWORDS

• Medical malpractice • Current issues

The underpinning of medical practice has always been patient care and patient safety. The past several decades, however, have seen an erosion of the patient-doctor relationship. Unfortunately, this erosion is caused by a variety of factors, including increased reliance on technology and pressure for increased clinical productivity. Added to this observation is the fact that the United States has become an increasingly litigious society with over 1,000,000 lawyers (approximately 1 per 300 citizens), which is far more than any other country. A number of factors have contributed to the ongoing medical malpractice crisis in the United States. There are three social goals of malpractice litigation: (1) to deter unsafe practices, (2) to compensate persons injured through negligence, and (3) to exact corrective justice.[1] This article examines how well the current system achieves these goals.

THE HISTORY

There have been three major medical malpractice crises in recent years in the United States.[2] The first occurred in the early to mid 1970s and was described as a crisis of insurance availability. Major malpractice insurers left the market and many physicians were unable to obtain coverage at any price. This gave rise to the formation of insurance companies owned and operated by physicians.

The second crisis in the early to mid 1980s was a crisis of affordability. Many physicians could not afford to pay the cost of increased premiums. The third and current crisis seems to involve both availability and affordability. Starting in 2001, there was an exodus of some of the larger malpractice carriers from the market. This has resulted in the inability of physicians to obtain malpractice insurance in some states and markedly increased the cost of insurance premiums in some areas. Some states, such as Florida, do not require physicians to carry liability insurance, which has resulted in an increasing number of physicians to "go bare" and not purchase insurance.[2] "Asset protection" is gaining increased attention by many physicians who decide not to purchase malpractice coverage.[2]

THE ROLE OF CAPS

Over the past several decades, as the malpractice crisis has intensified, there has been increasing focus on the impact of malpractice costs. The first major attempt at limiting caps was the California Medical Injury Compensation Reform Act (MICRA), which was passed in 1975. This legislation was passed in response to skyrocketing judgments in malpractice suits and dramatic increases in malpractice insurance premiums and decreased access to health care.[3] The malpractice environment in California at that time included a 200% increase in the number of malpractice claims in the preceding 10 years and a 1000% increase in the dollar amount of judgment awards in the prior decade. The major provisions of MICRA are listed in **Box 1**.[3] In California, since MICRA was enacted, benefits to the health care system have accrued. Specifically, lower malpractice premiums, improved patient access to care, and earlier and more equitable settlements have occurred since the passage of MICRA.[3] Malpractice caps

Department of Urology, Brigham and Women's Hospital, 45 Francis Street, ASB 11-3, Boston, MA 02115, USA
E-mail address: kloughlin@partners.org

Urol Clin N Am 36 (2009) 101–110
doi:10.1016/j.ucl.2008.08.006

alone have not proved, however, to be the panacea to the malpractice crisis that they were initially thought to be.

A cogent analysis of the impact of malpractice caps reveals there are multiple factors that influence physician premiums and the level of awards.[4] In the period between 1991 and 2002, the median payout in malpractice cases was 15.7% lower in states with caps compared with states without caps. Furthermore, during the same period, payouts increased by 83.3% in states with caps compared with 127.9% in states without caps. Despite these trends, however, there were unanticipated results. In states with caps the median annual premium increased by 48.2%, whereas in states without caps the annual premium increase was only 35.9%. The analysis by TheStreet.com Ratings concludes that there are other more important factors that drive up malpractice premiums than either caps or payout. They identify six other factors that influence medical malpractice premium rates (**Box 2**). These factors are reviewed next.

Box 2
Factors that influence medical malpractice premiums

1. The medical inflation rate
2. The insurance business cycle
3. The need to shore up insurance company reserves
4. A decline in investment income
5. Financial safety
6. Supply and demand

Data from TheStreet.comRatings. Accessed January 15, 2008.

The medical inflation rate continues significantly to outpace the national inflation rate. In 2005, total national health expenditures rose 6.9%, which was two times the rate of the inflation of the nation's economy.[5] This continued inflation influences malpractice awards where reimbursement for medical costs are considered.

The insurance business cycle is variable and cannot always be anticipated. When underwriting practices fail to cover anticipated claims this results in a shortfall for the insurers, which they react to by raising subsequent premiums.

Insurance company reserves are fluid and to a large degree unpredictable. When insurance companies write a new policy, they review previous claims experience, make some actuarial assumptions, and place a portion of that policy's premium into a reserve to cover expected future claims.[5] Most insurers make conservative assumptions when estimating reserves. If the assumptions err on the side of being overly optimistic, however, the level of reserves suffers and the only way to compensate for this misestimation is to raise future premiums.

Insurance companies make their profits not just by writing policies, but also by their investment income. When the stock market experiences a down period, the insurance companies can observe a dramatic decline in their investment income, which can be softened, in part, by raising premiums.

The financial corporations can also have an indirect impact on malpractice premiums. Insurance companies measure their financial strength based on evaluations of capitalization, reserve adequacy, profitability, liquidity, and stability.[5] If an analysis of these factors causes the directors of the corporation to conclude that their financial safety has been jeopardized, one remedy is to raise premiums.

The insurance industry, like other businesses, is influenced by the forces of supply and demand. The number of medical malpractice carriers has decreased over the past two decades and this has diminished somewhat the competition within the industry.

It should be clear that although caps on both economic and noneconomic damages may well have beneficial effects on lowering malpractice premiums, there are other forces that can have profound effects on the rates that insurance companies set on malpractice insurance. There are data to demonstrate, however, that caps have had some benefit in addressing the malpractice crisis. There is strong evidence that caps on noneconomic damages reduce the average size of awards by 20% to 30%.[6,7] There are also data to suggest that caps on noneconomic damages

Table 1
Medical malpractice liability reform summary

State	Punitive Damages	Noneconomic Damages
Alabama	—	—
Alaska	—	$400,000
Arizona	—	—
California	—	$250,000
Colorado	—	$1,000,000
Connecticut	—	—
Delaware	—	—
District of Columbia	—	—
Florida	$1,500,000	$1,000,000
Georgia	$250,000	—
Hawaii	—	$375,000
Idaho	$250,000	$250,000
Illinois	Not recoverable	—
Indiana	3 times compensatory damages or $50,000, whichever is greater	$250,000
Iowa	—	—
Kansas	The lesser of the defendant's annual gross income or $5,000,000	$250,000 from each party
Kentucky	—	—
Louisiana	Punitive damages prohibited at common law	$500,000 exclusive of future medical care
Maine	$75,000 in wrongful death	$400,000
Maryland	—	$500,000
Massachusetts	In wrongful death cases, not less than $5000 where punitive damages are appropriate; punitive damages otherwise prohibited at common law	$500,000
Michigan	Exemplary damages	$500,000
Minnesota	—	—
Mississippi	$20,000,000 if net worth greater than $1 billion, otherwise a sliding scale	$5,000,000
Missouri	—	$350,000 per defendant
Montana	—	$250,000
Nebraska	Punitive damages prohibited at common law	$1,750,000
Nevada	$300,000	$350,000
New Hampshire	No punitive damages in malpractice actions	$250,000
New Jersey	$350,000	—
New Mexico	—	$600,000
New York	—	—
North Carolina	$250,000	—
North Dakota	$250,000	$500,000
Ohio	—	$5000,000 for each plaintiff or $1,000,000 for each occurrence
Oklahoma	$500,000	$300,000

(continued on next page)

Table 1 (continued)		
State	**Punitive Damages**	**Noneconomic Damages**
Oregon	Prohibited against specified health practitioners	Felt to violate state constitution
Pennsylvania	When awarded, not less than $100,000	$1,500,000 per annual aggregate
Rhode Island	—	—
South Carolina	—	—
South Dakota	—	$500,000
Tennessee	—	—
Texas	$750,000	$250,000
Utah	—	$400,000 adjusted for inflation
Vermont	—	—
Virginia	$350,000	$1,500,000
Washington	Prohibited at common law	—
West Virginia	—	$250,000
Wisconsin	—	$350,000 or $500,000 if decreased minor
Wyoming	—	—

Data from Cohen H. Medical malpractice liability reform: legal issues and fifty-state survey of caps on punitive damages and noneconomic damages. CRS Reports for Congress, Washington, DC: Library of Congress; 4/11/05.

have a modest impact on premium growth. Recent studies show that caps have reduced the growth of premiums by 6% to 13%.[8,9]

Recent studies also suggest that state laws limiting malpractice awards have an impact on the geographic distribution of physicians. Encirosa and Hellinger[10] reported that between 1970 and 2000, the number of physicians per 100,000 residents more than doubled in the 13 states that enacted caps on noneconomic damages during the 1980s, compared with an 83% physician growth rate in the 23 states that did not cap malpractice awards before 2000. Further evidence of the beneficial effect of malpractice reforms was provided by Kessler and colleagues,[11] who reported a 3.3% increase in physician supply in states where such reforms were enacted. In some geographic areas the impact of malpractice reform is even greater. In Texas, in the 4 years since malpractice reform in 2003, medical license requests have increased by 18%.[12,13] A summary of medical malpractice liability reform appears in **Table 1**.

Not everyone is in agreement, however, that malpractice caps are worthwhile. The head of the Association of Trial Lawyers of America believes that caps set arbitrary, absolute limits on compensation and are unfair to patients. Some state courts have ruled that caps on awards to malpractice victims are unconstitutional.[14]

PATIENT SAFETY AND MEDICAL MALPRACTICE

Theoretically, one of the major goals of malpractice litigation should be to serve as an incentive to promote patient safety. The critical question is whether the current system achieves that goal. To answer that question, a research team at Harvard University reviewed the records from 30,000 hospital discharges and 3500 malpractice claims in New York State. They identified a rate of 3.7% adverse events and 1% negligent adverse events.[15] Overall there were 7.6 times as many negligent injuries as there were claims. Only 2% of negligent injuries resulted in claims and only 17% of claims seemed to involve a negligent injury.[16] A subsequent study conducted in Utah and Colorado in the late 1990s demonstrated almost identical results.[17] What explains this perverse discordance?

The start of the answer to that question began in November 1999 when the Institute of Medicine published its landmark treatise, "To Err Is Human: Building a Safer Health System." Aside from identifying different types of medical errors and

Box 3
American Urological Association guidelines for expert witness testimony in medical liability cases

The minimum qualification for expert witnesses should be the following:

1. Be active in the practice of urology at the time of the alleged occurrence.
2. Have current certification in urology from the American Board of Urology
3. Attain at least 5 years of practice after completing residency/fellowship training.
4. Be familiar with the applicable standard of care at the time of the alleged occurrence and with those books, journals, and other sources of information that establish the standard of care.

Additional standards established by the American Urological Association Board of Directors in October 2001 include:

- A urologist's review of the case should be complete and impartial.
- The expert witness should not be manipulated by an attorney into becoming an advocate or partisan for one side or another.
- The most objective testimony is that which could be used unaltered by either the defendant or the plaintiff.
- The urologist's testimony should help the court and jury to understand the standard of care in each situation and to distinguish between professional negligence and medical maloccurrence. These standards should not reflect the expert's personal bias, but should include all acceptable and realistic options for care as advocated by reputable and respected practicing urologists. Where possible, these standards should be in writing and should be evidence-based.
- The urologist should testify only about subject areas in which he or she is qualified by training and experience.
- An expert witness should not unduly profit from his or her consultation and testimony. Acceptance of compensation contingent upon the outcome of a case inconsistent with proper medical ethics.

Table 2
Malpractice claims in four countries, 2001

Country	Claims per 1000 Populations
United States	0.18
United Kingdom	0.12
Australia	0.12
Canada	0.04

Data from Anderson GF, Hussey PS, Frogner BK, et al. Health spending in the United States and the rest of the industrialized world. Health Aff 2005;24:903–14.

learn from errors. Clearly, under the present system, disclosure of any adverse event, whether or not negligence or malpractice is involved, exposes the provider to potential litigation. This culture undermines patient safety initiatives.

THE PHYSICIAN RESPONSE: DEFENSIVE MEDICINE

A natural response to an increased threat of litigation is to react defensively. Defensive medicine, however, is difficult to measure and identify. Nonetheless, in a mail survey to physicians in six high-risk specialties, 93% of respondents reported practicing defensive medicine.[18] The authors identified two categories of defensive medicine. The first was "assurance behavior," or ordering more diagnostic tests than were medically indicated. The second was "avoidance behavior," where high-risk patients are referred to other providers. Urologists are also affected by defensive medicine. A recent survey among urologists reported that 58% are considering referring difficult cases and 60% are considering limiting the scope of their practice.[19] In another survey of the New England Section of the American Urological Association,[20] 77% of the urologists polled affirmed that they practiced defensive medicine.

It is difficult to quantify the costs of defensive medicine because both assurance behavior and avoidance behavior are difficult to identify and measure. One study, however, estimated costs to be between $5 billion and $15 billion in 1991 dollars.[21] Current estimates by the US Department of Health and Human Services suggest that medical liability reforms would lead to a 5% to 9% decrease in medical expenses associated with defensive medicine. When these estimates are applied to the Federal Government, savings from reduced defensive medicine would range from $28.1 billion to $50.6 billion.

EXPERT WITNESSES

Any analysis of the malpractice crisis needs to examine the influence of expert witnesses in the litigation process. Although expert witnesses often

possible mechanisms of prevention, the report stated that acknowledgment and reporting of errors is essential for correction and prevention of future mistakes. One of the report's findings was that most errors are caused by faulty systems, processes, and conditions that lead people to make mistakes or fail to prevent them. The report also observed that many health care providers perceived the medical liability system as a serious impediment to systematic efforts to uncover and

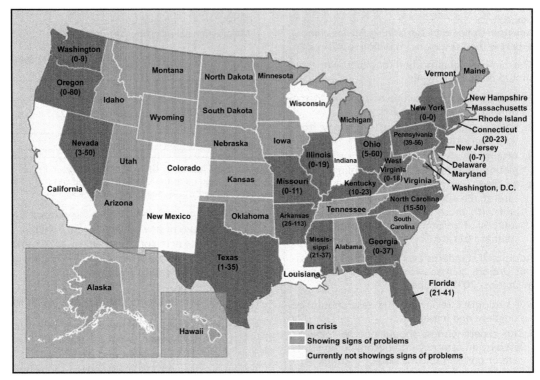

Fig. 1. Ranges of percentage increases in premiums between 2001 and 2002 for a standard professional liability insurance policy. (*From* Mello MM, Studdert DM, Brennan TA. The new medical malpractice crisis. N Engl J Med 2003;348(23):2281–4; with permission.)

play a pivotal role during medical malpractice cases, there are few objective standards as to what constitutes an expert. To ensure testimony that is a service to both the plaintiff and defendant, the American Urological Association has published standards for what constitutes expert urologic testimony. These guidelines appear in **Box 3**. These standards provide a foundation for expert testimony to be fair, impartial, and valuable during malpractice litigation. More subspecialty societies should provide such guidelines for their members and attorneys should select only credible experts to testify at trial.

THE CURRENT CRISIS

The current malpractice crisis continues unabated. Administrative costs (defense and underwriting costs) account for approximately 60% of total malpractice costs and only 50% of total malpractice costs are returned to patients.[22] The threat of litigation is ubiquitous and nationally there are more than 17 claims for every 100 full-time practicing physicians each year.[23] Compared with other nations, malpractice litigation in the United States is significantly more frequent. In the Unites States there are 50% more malpractice claims than in the Unites Kingdom and Australia and 450% more than in Canada (**Table 2**).[24]

These multiple forces, acting in concert, have caused the American Medical Association to identify 18 "crisis" states where physicians are having serious difficulties obtaining affordable professional liability insurance (**Fig. 1**).[2] **Tables 3** and **4** provide further data that compare the malpractice crisis by state.[25]

EXTENSION OF MALPRACTICE EXPOSURE

A recent ruling by the Supreme Judicial Court of Massachusetts provides the underpinning for the extension of malpractice vulnerability beyond the scope of the direct care of the patient. The court ruled that the mother of a boy who was hit by a car and died can sue the physician who prescribed medications to the driver, including narcotics, that can cause drowsiness. The court stated that the physician failed to warn the patient about the side effects of the medication and the potential danger of driving while taking them. The justice compared the role of the doctor with that of a bartender who serves a drink to a drunken customer.[26]

SOLUTIONS

The current malpractice litigation system is costly, not particularly efficient, and discourages the type

Table 3 Malpractice data by state: malpractice paid claims for 2003			
Rank		Paid Claims per 1000 Physicians[a]	Total Paid Claims
1	Indiana	30.5	423
2	Pennsylvania[b]	30.2	1249
3	Florida[b]	28.4	1261
4	Delaware	28	63
5	Montana	27.5	58
6	Wyoming[b]	24.6	24
7	Arizona	24.1	304
8	Louisiana	23.3	275
9	Nevada[b]	23.3	102
10	Kentucky[b]	23.1	219
11	New York[b]	22.9	1766
12	South Dakota	22.8	37
13	West Virginia[b]	22.8	105
14	Texas	22.3	1075
15	North Dakota	21.4	33
16	New Jersey[b]	20.1	585
17	Michigan	19.9	574
18	Mississippi[b]	19.5	103
19	Nebraska	19.5	83
20	Oklahoma	18.3	132
21	Rhode Island[b]	18.3	71
22	Utah	18.1	91
23	Iowa	18	116
24	Ohio[b]	17.9	577
25	Connecticut[b]	16.8	215
26	Georgia[b]	16.7	318
27	South Carolina	16.7	159
28	New Mexico	16.3	73
29	Kansas	16	102
30	Missouri[b]	14.7	225
31	California	14.1	1315
32	Alaska	13.6	19
33	Illinois[b]	13.6	491
34	Colorado	13.5	162
35	New Hampshire	13.5	47
36	Idaho	13.3	32
37	Maryland	13	280
38	Hawaii	12.7	48
39	Arkansas[b]	12.2	68
40	Washington	11.8	193
41	Oregon[b]	11.6	111
42	Vermont	11.5	26
43	District of Columbia	10.6	43

Table 3 (continued)			
Rank		Paid Claims per 1000 Physicians[a]	Total Paid Claims
44	Tennessee	10.3	156
45	North Carolina[b]	9.9	209
46	Maine	9.2	36
47	Virginia	9.2	182
48	Massachusetts[b]	8.8	250
49	Wisconsin	7.9	112
50	Minnesota	6.6	94
51	Alabama	5	48

[a] Includes active, nonfederal physicians.
[b] Currently on the AMA's list of malpractice crisis states.
Data from Kaiser Family Foundation. National practitioner data bank. May 2005. Available at: www.statechealthfacts.org/r/malpractice.cfm.

of disclosure that is paramount to improve patient safety. The cost of insurance coverage for hospital is usually linked to the history of claims from year to year, a process known as "experience rating."[2] Physicians, however, are typically not risk rated unless they have been repeatedly sued, in which circumstance they may have to obtain coverage from high-cost insurers or may not be able at all to get coverage.[27]

Studdert and colleagues[28] have outlined a series of proposals directed to improve the malpractice process. They have divided their proposals into tort reforms and system reforms, summarized in **Box 4**. The first group of tort reforms is directed at limitations on access to courts. Screening panels can be used to facilitate an evaluation of the merits of cases before they ever reach court. Another group of reforms is to shorten the statute of limitations (the period where a plaintiff can sue after discovering injury) or the statute of responses (the time of the actual negligent event rather than the time of discovery). Another category of tort reforms is the modification of liability rules. An example is eliminating joint-and-several liability, which means that a plaintiff may recover from multiple defendants only in proportion to their respective contributions to the causation of the injury. Another reform is the elimination of the doctrine of res ipsa loquitor, which establishes a new standard for expert witnesses. An additional reform is to enforce higher standards for proving breaches of informed consent.

A third category of tort reforms is aimed at limiting the size of awards. These reforms place caps

Table 4
Malpractice data by state: average malpractice payments in 2003

Rank		Average Payment ($)
1	Hawaii	501,161
2	Illinois[a]	494,857
3	Connecticut[a]	486,759
4	District of Columbia	428,081
5	Massachusetts[a]	407,441
6	New York[a]	380,000
7	Nevada[a]	379,578
8	Georgia[a]	370,691
9	Minnesota	353,201
10	Arkansas[a]	352,397
11	Montana	348,448
12	Oklahoma	342,451
13	Rhode Island[a]	341,254
14	Ohio[a]	340,734
15	North Carolina[a]	333,008
16	Oregon[a]	324,788
17	New Jersey[a]	322,392
18	Alaska	311,842
19	Maryland	310,551
20	West Virginia[a]	309,543
21	Florida[a]	309,236
22	Pennsylvania[a]	305,704
23	Arizona	297,332
24	Indiana	296,819
25	Virginia	288,578
26	Mississippi[a]	285,209
27	South Dakota	266,486
28	Tennessee	266,255
29	Wisconsin	261,545
30	South Carolina	256,179
31	Idaho	253,383
32	Missouri[a]	252,949
33	New Hampshire	247,872
34	Colorado	245,687
35	Washington	241,522
36	Texas	225,403
37	Alabama	225,199
38	Delaware	223,472
39	Iowa	217,759
40	Maine	214,236
41	Kentucky[a]	211,039
42	Wyoming[a]	207,531
43	Nebraska	193,355

Table 4
(continued)

Rank		Average Payment ($)
44	Kansas	190,331
45	North Dakota	189,561
46	California	172,626
47	Louisiana	171,927
48	New Mexico	149,606
49	Vermont	137,346
50	Michigan	130,945
51	Utah	125,924

[a] Currently on the AMA's list of malpractice crisis states.
Data from Kaiser Family Foundation. National practitioner data bank. May 2005. Available at: www.statehealthfacts.org/r/malpractice.cfm.

on either total damages or "pain and suffering" damages. In addition, there have been proposals to limit the contingency fees of attorneys, which are typically in the range of 30% to 40% of the settlement. Other reforms directed at reducing the size of payments are "collateral source offsets" and "periodic payments." Collateral source offsets prevent plaintiffs from recovering losses that can be recouped from other sources, such as health insurance. Periodic payments prevent the plaintiff from receiving the award in a lump sum, but rather receive payments installments as the expenditures arise.

The other group of proposals recommended by Studdert and colleagues[28] is directed at a fundamental reform of the system. One approach is an early offer program where there are incentives to litigants to arrive at a private settlement soon after an adverse event occurs.[29] Other alternatives include arbitration through mediation or medical courts.[30]

Another approach to reform of the system is to eliminate negligence as the basis of eligibility for compensation, as is the standard in workers' compensation cases. This system identifies clinical outcomes that, by their very nature, are likely to be preventable and then facilitate speedy compensation.[31]

A final alternative is the so-called "enterprise-liability models" where the enterprise, in many cases the hospital or health maintenance organization, assumes primary responsibility for any patient injury. The liability costs vary annually based on the enterprise's overall injury experience. This type of system emphasizes the value of systematic approaches to quality improvement.

Box 4
Malpractice reform options

Tort reform

Limitations on access to courts

    Establish screening panels

    Shorten statute of limitations

    Shorten statute of responses

Modification of liability rules

    Eliminate joint and several liability rules

    Impose higher standards for breaches of informed consent

    Eliminate res ipsa loquitor

Damages reform

    Cap damages

    Limit attorney fees

    Mandate collateral source offsets

    Mandate periodic payments

System reform

Alternative mechanisms for resolving disputes

    Encourage early offers for settlements

    Medical courts

    Compensation through a fault-based system

Alternative to the negligence standard

    Compensation through a no-fault system

    Implement predesignated compensable events

Relocation of legal responsibility

    Enterprise liability (shift responsibility from individuals to organizations)

Data from Studdert DM, Mello MM, Brennan TA. Medical malpractice. N Engl J Med 2004;350:283–92; with permission.

IMPROVING THE PERFORMANCE OF ATTORNEYS, JUDGES, AND JURIES

Not all lawyers are adept at assessing the validity of a potential malpractice case. Some states have instituted "certificate of merit requirements," which mandate that a plaintiff's lawyer must consult a medical expert at the outset to help filter out unsubstantial claims. Another alternative that has not been adequately explored is to require the legal profession to develop a system to measure proficiency, such as routinely done in the medical profession. At present, there is no mechanism whereby a trial lawyer must demonstrate a proficiency in medical malpractice litigation. Such a requirement could potentially prevent less-skilled attorneys from overloading the system with cases of little or no merit. Better trained attorneys with a special expertise in malpractice litigation are more likely to judge which cases should be settled before going to trial.

In addition to the continued training of attorneys, the ongoing education of judges has, in some cases, been underserved. Struve[32] has advocated that states adopt a "continuing judicial education" program that trains judges in case management skills and equips judges to be better able to assess the qualifications of medical, statistical, and economic experts.

Juries ultimately decide the outcome of any malpractice trial. Legal scholars have debated several provisions that may make the task of the jurors easier. One proposal is to allow jurors to take notes during testimony. Proponents assert that note taking would help jurors recall relevant evidence, whereas skeptics claim it would prove to be a distraction. This needs to be more thoroughly investigated.

Another proposal is to give judges the discretion to permit questioning of witnesses by jurors. In such an arrangement, the judge would instruct the jurors that they can pose factual or clarifying questions by submitting the questions, in writing, before the witness is excused. The jury would be told in advance that the judge will discuss each question with counsel, privately, before deciding whether to pose it and that the jurors should not draw any conclusions whether the judge decides whether or not to ask a particular question.[32]

THE PERFECT STORM

The current malpractice system is costly, inefficient, and in many cases unfair. Major reforms are urgently needed to achieve the goal of all parties involved: to improve the quality of patient care.

At the same time that the patient safety movement is gaining increasing momentum, the public's frustration with the medical and legal professions is increasing. This confluence of factors may result in the perfect storm to achieve what all parties are seeking: better care for everyone.

REFERENCES

1. Keeton WP, Dobbs DB, Keeton RE, et al. Prosser and Keeton on the law of torts. 5th edition. St. Paul (MN): West Publishing; 1984.
2. Mello MM, Studdert DM, Brennan TA. The new medical malpractice crisis. N Engl J Med 2003;348(23):2281–4.

3. Available at: www.thedoctors.com/advocacy/miora. asp. Accessed January 15, 2008.

4. Available at: www.TheStreet.comRatings. Accessed January 15, 2008.

5. Catli AC, Cowan C, Heffler S, et al. National health spending in 2005. Health Aff 2006;26(1):142–53.

6. Danzon PM. The frequency and severity of medical malpractice claims: new evidence. Law Contemp Probl 1986;49(2):57–84.

7. Sloan FA, Morgenhagen PM, Boubjerg RR. Effects of tort reforms on the value of closed medical malpractice claims: a microanalysis. J Health Polit Policy Law 1989;14(4):663–89.

8. Thorpe KE. The medical malpractice crisis: recent trends and the impact of state tort reforms. Health Aff, Supplement Web Exclusive, Jan–June 2004.

9. Danzon PM, Epstein AJ, Johnson S, et al. The crisis in medical malpractice insurance. In: Harris R, Litan R, editors. Brookings-Wharton papers on financial services. Washington, DC: Brookings Institution Press; 2004.

10. Encinosa WE, Hellinger FJ. Have state caps on malpractice awards increased the supply of physicians? Health Aff (Jan-June 2005) Suppl Web Exclusive W5-250–8.

11. Kessler DP, Sage WM, Becker DA. Impact of malpractice reforms on the supply of physician services. JAMA 2005;293(21):2618–25.

12. New York Times, Oct. 4, 2007.

13. Mehlman M. Promoting fairness in the medical malpractice system. In: Sage WM, Kersh R, editors. Medical malpractice and the U.S. health care system. Cambridge (UK): Cambridge University Press; 2006. p. 37–153.

14. Forster S. State's high court lifts caps on pain, suffering awards. Milwaukee Journal Sentinel July 15, 2005.

15. Harvard Medical Practice Study. Patients, doctors, and lawyers: medical injury, malpractice litigation and patient compensation in New York: report of the Harvard Medical Practice Study to the state of New York. Cambridge (MA): President and Fellows of Harvard College; 1990.

16. Localio AR, Lawthers AG, Brennan TA, et al. Relation between malpractice claims and adverse events due to negligence: results of the Harvard Medical Practice Study III. N Engl J Med 1991;325:245–51.

17. Thomas EJ, Studdert DM, Burstin HR, et al. Incidence and types of adverse events and negligent care in Utah and Colorado. Med Care 2000;38:261–71.

18. Studdart DM, Mello MM, Sage WM, et al. Defensive medicine among high-risk specialist physicians in a volatile malpractice environment. JAMA 2005; 293(21):2609–17.

19. Sobel DL, Loughlin KR, Cougan CL. Medical malpractice liability in clinical urology: a survey of practicing urologists. J Urol 2006;175:1847–51.

20. New England section of the American Urological Association: Highlighter-Special edition, 2007 Member Survey Results.

21. Robin RJ, Mendelson DN. How much does defensive medicine cost? J Am Health Policy 1994; 4:7–15.

22. Kakalik JS, Pace N. Costs and compensation paid in tort litigation. Santa Monica (CA): RAND; 1986.

23. Anderson RE. Billions for defense the pervasive nature of defensive medicine. Arch Intern Med 1999; 159:2399–402.

24. Anderson GF, Hussey PS, Frogner BK, et al. Health spending in the United States and the rest of the industrialized world. Health Aff 2005;24(4): 903–14.

25. Rice B. Where does your state rank? Med Econ 2005;82(19):72, 74–5.

26. Kowalczyk L. SJC ruling adds to doctor liability. Boston Globe; December 11, 2007:B1.

27. Schwartz WB, Mendelsohn DN. Physician who have lost their malpractice insurance: their demographic characteristics and the surplus-lines companies that insure them. JAMA 1989;262: 1335–41.

28. Studdert DM, Mello MM, Brennan TA. Medical malpractice. N Engl J Med 2004;350(3):283–92.

29. O'Connell J. Offers that can't be refused: foreclosure of personal injury claims by defendants' prompt tender of claimants net economic losses. Northwest Univ Law Rev 1982;77:589–632.

30. Johnson KB, Phillips CG, Orentlicher D, et al. A fault based administrative alternative for resolving medical malpractice claims. Vanderbilt Law Rev 1989; 42:1365–406.

31. Bovbjerg RR, Tancredi LB, Gaylin DS. Obstetrics and malpractice: evidence on the performance of a selective no-fault system. JAMA 1991;265: 2836–43.

32. Struve CT. Expertise and the legal process. In: Sage WM, Kersh R, editors. Medical malpractice and the U.S. health care system. Cambridge (UK): Cambridge University Press; 2006. p. 173–90.

Index

Note: Page numbers of article titles are in **boldface** type.

Urol Clin N Am 36 (2009) 111–114
doi:10.1016/S0094-0143(08)00133-X
0094-0143/08/$ – see front matter © 2008 Elsevier Inc. All rights reserved.

urologic.theclinics.com

Printed and bound by CPI Group (UK) Ltd, Croydon, CR0 4YY

03/10/2024

01040361-0009